PREPARED!

A Healthcare Guide for Aging Adults

Written by Cheryl Field, MSN, RN, CRRN

"Cheryl Field has created an invaluable tool for individuals who could use a hand navigating through the incredibly complex world of healthcare as an older adult."

- James M. Berklan | Executive Editor McKnight's Long-Term Care News

ISBN: 978-1-960136-30-5

Dedication

Prepared! A Healthcare Guide for Aging Adults

This book is dedicated to all those humans who embraced me as their "nurse". Some for just a little while, others for longer periods of time. Each of you taught me something about the human condition, the importance of vulnerability, trust, and empathy for one another. In every word, sentence, and chapter, the echoes of your lives reverberate, leaving an everlasting mark on the soul of this book.

Most prominent in my memories are days spent as an advocate, caregiver, and daughter for my mother, Ethel Patricia Diamond. The last few months of her life in 2009 planted the seeds for his work. Those seeds grew into a system of ideas, and behaviors for advocates everywhere to leverage while supporting loved ones on their healthcare journey.

This work culminated in 2020 as the world was facing a global pandemic it did not know was coming, our family was facing the end of life for Marguerite "Chum" Sholik. Most of us believe we have a guardian angel, I was lucky to live with mine. Chum made it possible for me to travel and teach others, while raising a family. I last saw her 4 days before she passed, I had travel booked which I contemplated canceling. She told me "Go! Get your work done!" Her photo graces the cover of Prepared! A Healthcare Guide for Aging Adults. It is the work she meant for me to finish.

Table of Contents

Introduction

The phone rings at 3:00 AM and wakes you from a deep sleep. Instantly you know it's the call you feared, and it's actually happening. For us living with an aging parent next door, the call we feared happened frequently. This time it was 3:00 AM and we were awakened by the life alert operator.

"Your aunt has fallen, she's able to speak to us. She's in pain but said she did not want us to call 911; she did not want to wake up 'the kids'. She says she wants you to come over. Can you go over to her house now?" the Life Alert operator asked us calmly. With a dry mouth and a noticeable lump in my throat I replied in a whisper at first, "Yes". Then louder, " Yes, it will only take a minute," I replied into the phone. My husband is now awake as well as asking questions. " What's going on? Is she okay?" he asked me as I strained to hear the 911 operator, willing my face not to show my internal panic. It's hard not to panic. His aunt had lived with us for 10 years, and she had fallen many times. This was not the first nor last call we would be awakened to. She was only a flight of stairs and an interior door away, but it felt like an eternity from the moment the phone rang to the moment we would arrive at her side.

"It will only take one minute." I had reassured the Life Alert operator. Quietly making my way down the steps felt like an hour. My thoughts raced with questions, "Would she be bleeding? What if she broke something? What if she was really hurt this time? How will our kids react?" Fear, panic, and uncertainty all flooded my mind in that one minute. Then I'm there with her and I know we are going to need help, which means asking the Life Alert operator to dispatch to 911. Calling for an ambulance in a small town at 3:00 AM means waking up volunteers and waiting for them to drive from their personal homes to the Volunteer Fire Department where they will suit up and get into their rigs and turn on their alarms and come with their piercing sirens in the quiet of night to our home. So for now I'm the first responder. I think *It's okay I'm a nurse. I have to be OK, right?* Well I'm not an emergency room nurse but for now I'm the only nurse that's here. I'm it, I'm here with her and for the next 15 minutes that's all she has.

I'm volleying back and forth in my heart and head. *What am I going to need to communicate with the ambulance and the hospital personnel? They don't know her at all.* Think, think, think… ID and her insurance card, a medication list, a diagnosis list, glasses, dentures or partials, and her hearing aid. Once she gets evaluated in the hospital, if they determine she has to be admitted, there might be a trip to a rehabilitation facility, and that will require sweatpants and clothing and crossword puzzle books, reading glasses, her favorite brush and hair pick. I know she does not want to go to the hospital, and I wonder how long it might be before she's able to get back home. I wonder who will advocate for her and her needs in a new healthcare system? Will there be anyone we know there? What will happen if she can't return to her home with us? There are many questions which pulse through my mind as I drive to the hospital. As prepared as I thought I was then, I had not read this book, and I was not completely prepared.

Does any of this sound familiar? It's a common starting place in the unexpected and undesired journey into the healthcare system for hospitalization and after hospitalization service utilization. This book is written for aging adults and their family members to replace the fear and uncertainty with calm and confidence.

Prepared: A Healthcare Guide for Aging Adults promises to simply and swiftly arm individuals and family members with strategies and tactics for not only surviving but thriving through the transitions brought on by changes in health status. This can be an overwhelming time in you or your loved ones life, so to bring your instant sense of "you got this" I'm going to teach you to bring your own B.I.T.C.H. This is a funny, provocative, and easy to remember framework for you or your loved ones to follow. B.I.T.C.H.

Capital B stands for the **Be Prepared** for that "Oh Sh*t" moment when there is a change in your health status and it's time for you to bring it! Bring what you might ask? This book starts with walking you through how to get prepared for an "Oh Sh*t" moment. You will learn exactly what to bring and how to be prepared.

Capital I represents **Information.** A well-informed consumer of healthcare services is the very best "patient" and will have the most success leveraging the healthcare system to reach their individual goals. At each stage of transition we will outline the questions to ask, so you gain the information you need and add to your growing knowledge base.

Capital T represents **Taking** control. Leveraging the information and aligning that with your health goals for you or your loved ones will be instrumental in contributing to the overall plan of care set forth by the healthcare team. This makes sure that you are driving the direction and making the decisions around the care services you choose to undergo in order to achieve your optimal health outcomes.

Capital C stands for **Communication** and the essential function that communication plays in making sure the right information and plan for care will ensure your desired health outcomes. Communication between key parties such as the patient, the provider, and the payer will prove to be essential in care coordination. Continuity of care demands consistent data flow and communication can, and must, fill in gaps of poor data flow.

H stands for **Home** and the planning and steps taken to move from inpatient and institutional care settings to alternative care settings, which may be back to your old home or to a new alternative home.

What you are holding in your hands are years of lessons learned as both a professional nurse working in senior care, and as a caregiver, daughter, sister, and friend slimmed down into easy to follow advice. The objective for completing this work was to give readers a self-guided advocacy book to be used again and again. Documenting advice, tips, and suggestions in small doses of content, based on where you or your loved ones journey or specific point of transition in and out of the healthcare system. A guide book to help reduce the feelings of fear and uncertainty and replace them with calm and confidence.

Why should you read this book? Written by a nurse with 30+ years experience in the healthcare setting and formal education through a Master's Degree in Adult Ambulatory Care, and edited by nurse colleagues, *Prepared: Mastering Transition for Seniors* will provide you with expert "insider's" advice which will serve as a resource to come back to again and again. Throughout this book, you will find personal and professional stories and lessons learned, summary tips, and resource materials. Beyond the stories are facts and resources for those of you who wish to go beyond this book and make it easy for you to put the right words into your internet search engine to get the answers that you're looking for. This book will prepare you for the unexpected, yet highly expected "Oh Sh*t" moments that are undesired, and yet become a reality for many of us in the later years in life. With age comes change, let's get you prepared!

Part One: Being Prepared for an "Oh Sh*t" Moment

What is this moment I call the "Oh Sh*t" moment? Maybe you or a loved one has fallen, or experienced a sudden onset of new pain, a loss in a normal ability, or the realization that a loved one might be nearing the end of life. *Something dramatic has changed.* You find yourself feeling panicked, filled with uncertainty, and by being caught up in the moment you feel completely out of control. You might be thinking "Oh sh*t now what do I do?" Okay right there - as if this were a movie let's push the pause button. An emergent situation is upon you- what do you do now? I have asked myself that question many times, and I found answers that made a difference, and it is exactly why I wrote this book. As a nurse who worked nearly 15 years on the front line in hospital and nursing homes, I share my expertise throughout these pages. This book is for everyone over 50; none of us want to think about a sudden change in health, and we all need to! being unprepared for events which do happen, for example a serious car accident, can send you or your loved one into the healthcare system without an informed advocate. Imagine if this happened to my husband, and the ER nurse asked me what medications my husband was taking. As I write this sentence, I have to admit I could not answer that question specifically. I am facing the need to get prepared for an "Oh Sh*t" moment just like you. We are in this together. I have a unique perspective as an insider from the healthcare industry, and as a consumer of healthcare services, so I know how both the nurse and the family think, act, and feel. *Prepared!* will guide you. You will know what to do, what to ask, and what you might feel as well. This book is like having a remote control, you can push pause, gather what you need, and be ready for the next scene when you push play. Remember, an emergency has occurred and you are wondering what to do next. Let's push the play button. In an emergency most will call 911, and at that time you immediately transfer trust and confidence to the operator who will stay on the phone until a first responder arrives. The kind face of an emergency medical technician who enters your home, offers reassurance, and seemingly takes over at a time when making any decisions at all feels impossible. This was your "Oh Sh*t" moment.

These moments happen and I want you or your loved one to be ready for them. I don't want to simplify or underestimate the amount of impact these moments can have in your life, but let's for a moment think of it like a fire drill. When the fire alarm goes off, you have to know what to do in order to successfully and safely exit the building and know that everyone is out of the building. As a result, there are procedures that we follow in a fire drill, and it's important that we actually practice these procedures. Nobody wants to think about this moment. I'm here to tell you that you have to if you want to safely and successfully "exit the building". Being prepared everyday requires you to take some proactive steps. This work requires some pre-planning and I admit these are not necessarily items any of us want on our to do list. You are reading this book, which tells me you are ready to get prepared. Good for you!

You might be reading this book because your parent or spouse is getting older, and you are worried an "Oh Sh*t" moment or two are in your future. Maybe your parent(s) or spouse are not a planner; YOU ARE, and that's great news for you and your loved one! Whether you are reading this book to help get your friend, spouse, or parent(s) prepared or are trying to get your siblings to face the need for some preparation and planning as your own parents age, this book is written for **all of you**. You are investing time to become an informed healthcare advocate. The return on that investment will be realized as you navigate more confidently through the healthcare system. There are a few areas you need to work through to be prepared. Keep going, you got this!

Being Prepared With Medications:

Medications: The goal of this preparation step is to keep a current list of all the medications you put in your body every day. This will include those medications that you need a prescription for and those medications you take that you can buy without a prescription, called over the counter. Your body is one massive chemistry lab, and any additional chemicals going in are of great importance to communicate. Knowing what goes in your body will serve you well, especially when changes to those medications happen. We will talk more about that in later chapters.

You will notice in the healthcare system there is an emphasis on medication review. Insiders call this a "medication reconciliation" and it has become one of the topmost important review processes that all healthcare providers are taking. So much so that you may even get a little bored of reviewing your own medications with practitioners. You'll also feel frustrated when you realize that the electronic medical record system of the practitioner that you are sitting in front of is old and outdated and may not have all of your current medications properly listed. This will become obvious to you when you are in the emergency room in the hospital or even in an outpatient physician office or a pre-surgical care center. Each person you come in contact with is going to ask you to review your list of medications.

Medications can be confusing based on the fact that the name that you know the medication by may be different from what the medication is listed as in the electronic medical record system. Just like people have names at birth then nicknames that get assigned over years or shortened versions of your original name, the same can be true of medication names which change even though it's still the same medication. When a drug is first put onto the market, it is given a formal name called the "brand name" that protects the drug manufacturer for a number of years before people can begin to copy the recipe of that drug. Once the drug has been on the market for a number of years, it can be copied legally and you might start to see a different name that we refer to as the "trade or generic name" of that drug. Then there's also the name you give your medication like your "pee pill" or your "heart pill" that you come to know them as, and you've long forgotten either the brand or the trade name of the medication.

It's helpful to keep a list of your medication using all of these names, the brand, the trade or generic, and how you refer to it and even a list of the description of the pill. Some manufacturers make the pill in a light pink color while other manufacturers might make the exact same medication in a slightly different color. That can be confusing when you are admitted into an institution, and they present to you what doesn't look familiar and tell you that it's the medication you've always taken at home.

Let me give you a couple of examples. Tylenol is also called Acetaminophen; it's generally taken for mild to moderate pain like a headache. The extra strength 500 mg tablet is an oblong white tablet which is what I take, and I always take 2 at a time for headache. Ibuprofen, which is a non-steroidal anti-inflammatory drug also used for mild to moderate pain, helps me when my arthritis is bothering me and I feel stiffness in my joints. You might know this drug by its brand names like Motrin (US market) or Actiprofen (Canadian market). Both Tylenol and Ibuprofen would be on my medication list with all the details. Now let's add into the example a high-risk medication like coumadin, a commonly prescribed blood thinner. Also known as Warfarin, this medication is used to treat blood clots, or prevent blood clots from forming in your body. Your daily dose can vary, and your blood needs to be monitored to make sure the medication is not having too much impact on your body's ability to form a clot, resulting in bleeding. Below is what my medication list might look like, including my latest blood work in the comments.

Generic Name	Brand Name	Dose	Frequency	Why I take it	Last taken	Details/ Labs
Acetaminophen	Tylenol	500 mg	as needed	headache	8/21/2023	
Ibuprofen	Motrin	200 mg	as needed	joint pain	7/15/2023	
Warfarin	Coumadin or Jantoven	2.5 mg	Daily	to prevent clots due to my abnormal heart rhythm	8/21/2023	Protime 2.5 add date
Covid 19 vaccine	Pfizer Covid 19 vaccine	1 shot	every 6 months	prevent serious infection	5/16/2023	

To be prepared in the B.I.T.C.H framework you must know the drugs that you put into your body every day, what they are for, and be able to identify them at least based on how you've taken them at home. Record the time of day you usually take your medications, and for medications taken weekly, or monthly. Note the date of your last dose. This is very helpful. Vaccinations or immunizations should also be listed in the same place. Vaccinations to prevent shingles, flu, pneumonia, and Covid are becoming a focus in adult care. Keeping track of the date of these vaccinations and having that record accessible to you or your loved one in case of an emergency makes life easier.

You'll find a resource section on my website www.cherylfield.com where you can download a medication schedule and fill in all this data. When you fill up your medication "pill box" each week or two, review this list and note any changes that might have occurred from week to week. Keep a current medication card ready to go in case an "Oh Sh*t" moment was to occur. Keep in mind these moments are not scheduled- we don't know when they're coming,and you must be prepared!

Being Prepared With Past Surgeries and Medical Conditions

In addition to medication, you should keep a list of your past surgeries and any other treatments or procedures you have had in the past, along with the location, the provider, and the date. Again, this information is often inaccurate and incomplete in any one of the electronic medical records of the many providers that you may see. At the time of publication in 2023, all healthcare networks are not yet connected and sharing data across them. While it seems shocking that one can order a product on the Internet and have it delivered nearly instantaneously or at least by the next day, ironically, healthcare information is still challenged by disconnected networks of care providers and nonstandard data exchange. There are investments and efforts being made to connect networks, but we are not all there yet. There is key information you should carry in order to ensure that wherever you are within the healthcare network, the information you bring is accurate and up to date so that you can share with every provider.

It is very helpful to give the healthcare provider who is assisting you through this "Oh Sh*t" moment a list of similar past moments that you have experienced. Imagine if you have had multiple surgeries, original parts of your body modified, implants put in, or other items removed. As a care provider you're trying to evaluate that person, but you don't know all of the changes that have occurred since birth. I can make a guess that you have all of your original parts and they're all working and there haven't been any modifications to them; however, having a list of past surgeries, treatments, and procedures takes the guesswork out of that. Further, it actually informs that care provider on what to expect when they begin to help figure out what is going on with your health that has resulted in bringing you into the healthcare system urgently. This is also recommended to be written down, and put on your refrigerator, and updated again each time you visit the doctor. If you have a new treatment or procedure you should update the list. Many doctor's offices have tools for listing past treatments and surgeries, you can use an index card, or make a note in your phone notes app. If you are looking for more check out the resources tab on my website www.cherylfield.com; there are links to more tools for getting prepared with past medical history.

Being Prepared With Advance Directives and Other Instructional Documents

The third important component of information that you will be asked about will be regarding advance directives and any end of life decisions which you may have made with your healthcare proxy or in advance of this moment. Again, a topic very few of us really want to think about that becomes quite essential in an emergency situation when healthcare providers are just trying to do for you what you want done for yourself. If you don't have written down advance directives and are reading this book, you should add this to your To-Do List before you move to the next chapter.

You can get started easily on this topic. If you Google advance directives you can get a printable form that you can fill out before you finish the cup of coffee in your hand. There are two main elements in an advance directive—*a living will and a durable power or health care proxy* depending on your state. There are also other documents that can supplement your advance directive. You can choose which documents to create, depending on how you want decisions to be made. Links for state specific documents can be found on my website www.cherylfield.com under the resource tab. No matter what your state calls these forms, the goal is to communicate in writing your wishes and separately identify a person other than yourself who would be responsible for assuring your instructions are executed. The time to prepare is now, so you remain in control even if you are not able to speak for yourself.

Be sure to communicate your wishes in your current health network by sharing a copy of the document with your primary care doctor, the hospitals and clinics you would most likely frequent, and your person who will speak on your behalf. Keep a copy or two on hand in an envelope and attach it to the refrigerator or place it in a folder on the back of your front entry door. My third grade teacher and lifelong friend keeps his advance directives on a flash drive in his pocket everyday! The format you chose does not matter. The goal is to have these key instructions available to first responders in an emergency situation. I have been involved in too many personal and professional situations where the healthcare team lacks the content of an advance directive. No provider wants to perform cardiopulmonary resuscitation or CPR on a patient who had been found in cardiac arrest only to later discover that the patient did not want CPR in the event of a cardiac arrest. Communicating your wants and wishes gives you control even when you're in a situation medically where you're not able to be in control.

As mentioned in the introduction the capital "C" in B.I.T.C.H. stands for communication and this is essential for continuity of care and you own the responsibility of clearly communicating what it is that you want. So spend some time on the website or sit with a family member who might review the website with you if you don't already have advance directives in place. If you take this one action step, you will be on your way to being prepared!

Being Prepared With Usual Day to Day Activities and Capabilities

I want to talk about your usual day-to-day activities. Although this may not seem as interesting or intriguing or important to you, it is really helpful when you can communicate your abilities, and your needs. Hospital staff will look at "you" and see their own biased "older person". They will make assumptions, and act on these assumptions. You might not have your glasses and hearing aids with you, making communication impossible. They might label you confused when in fact you simply cannot hear. In Part Two the importance of a good description of your prior level of function and continued service delivery in a rehabilitation stay is reviewed.

Think about your usual day: how you normally wake up, what time of day that is at, what your normal routine is for bathing, dressing, and your first meal of the day. Do you normally put on the television or do you like music; is it quiet? Is there a tablet you like to use to read the morning news? This is not the time for you to think about and record your ideal day, this is about your *usual* day, what really happens. For me on an ideal day I might go for a five-mile run, but on a usual day I walk about 50 feet to my office and begin work and skip the gym all together. You get my point. This is a time to be honest and give the care providers around you an understanding of how much you're able to do for yourself on a normal day and how much assistance you need over the course of a day or a week or even a month.

Many of you are completely independent and you are able to wake in the morning, get out of bed alone, and prepare for the day with personal hygiene like taking a shower, brushing your teeth, preparing food, moving, etc. Others may find that their "activities of daily living", as they're known in the healthcare world, require assistance from other people and/or the use of assistive devices in order to achieve those things independently. Do you use glasses and hearing aids, dentures and/or long handled reachers, scooters, golf carts etc.? Frankly, I still drive my car to the grocery store and am quite dependent on my car as an assistive device to efficiently, safely, and physically get to the grocery store and return to home. So think about these assistive devices as items that you use to get the job done.

On my website www.cherylfield.com you will find a form for recording your usual activities of daily living. You can record your normal and usual activities of daily living along with any assistive devices or assistance from others that you receive throughout the day, week, or month. Updating this list gives you and any future caregivers the detailed information they need. Have it ready in the event that caregivers or first responders urgently enter your home.

As you are evaluating your usual activities it is imperative that you consider how you access help in the event of an emergency. There are many different monitoring services ranging from traditional providers like Life Alert to new technologies embedded in smart watches. The key is to make sure that you or your loved one can access help should an emergency situation occur while they are home alone.

Being Prepared to Communicate Your Pain

Pain is so central to how we are as humans and its impact on our whole being should not be overlooked. Your care providers will need to learn from you about any pain you experience. Pain is highly subjective; it is only you who can describe your pain, making it a challenging area of clinical assessment to document. To help standardize the assessment, process clinicians use a 10-point pain scale where zero is no pain and 10 is the worst pain. Have you thought about your pain this way? At what point in your pain experience do you seek interventions? Do you rely on non-medication based interventions like stretching, yoga, mindfulness, aromatherapy, etc.? Write this down. Do you have success managing your pain with medications? When you take those medications, how long before you typically experience pain relief? I also like to think about pain which interferes with function and pain but does not interfere with function and can be tolerated. Spending a little time being able to know and describe the usual amount of pain you experience while functioning is important. Is there pain which you experience which is so severe that you simply do not do that activity, or does the pain hold you back from enjoying certain activities? There are links to tools you might find helpful at www.cherylfield.com in the resource tab on pain assessments.

Doing this pain awareness work as part of the preparation phase will serve you should you find yourself in an inpatient setting where you are not freely accessing your own medication bottles. Many doctors prescribe pain medications to be given based on the pain scale score described by the patient. So your pain medication orders might say one tablet of pain medication, for example Percocet, for pain between one and five as reported by the patient or two tablets if six or higher. When a nurse asks you about your pain, they should describe the pain scale being used and ask you to rate your pain before they dispense your medications. You might find that you experience a lot of pain in therapy and want to be proactive in taking your medications. This will require advocacy. Asking about how the medications are ordered before you experience any pain is very helpful for you to establish if the orders are going to meet your pain management needs. We will cover this topic again in the skilled nursing and rehabilitation section.

Being Prepared for Updates

Now that you have all of the documents on the fridge, keep your heart and mind open to the fact that things may change. As you enter and exit the healthcare system you will want to update those changes and do your best to always have a most recent copy of these documents in an envelope, out in the open (which is why I suggest an envelope and a big magnet on the side of your fridge). Some of these documents are going to change very rarely. For example, your advance directives will most often stay the same; however, you may find that your medication list changes frequently. You can have access to blank documents at my website www.cherylfield.com under the resources tab. Print them anytime you need a new copy to update with changes. Bravo for getting this far!

Part Two: Thriving on the Inside of Healthcare Institutions

Congratulations on taking the time to get prepared for an unexpected future event. Some of you are reading part two as a proactive step to get yourself educated just in case something happens - that is a great investment! For others, you are doubling back since you last read this section. An unexpected change has occurred and you or your loved one is now entering the healthcare system with uncertainty and admittedly some fear. This section will educate you and provide expert guidance. I include suggested question lists, tips to help you to think about what's next, and provide resources for when you want more help. Read it as many times as you need every time you find yourself back in this state I call a "vulnerable transition state" as the result of an "Oh Sh*t" moment.

No Matter the Healthcare Setting These Matters Matter!

In this section I want to give you an insider's perspective on something very important: the business that exists within healthcare. It does not matter which part of the healthcare system you are receiving services from, there are a few themes they all have in common. First, we must acknowledge healthcare in the US is a business and the providers of services need to collect payments to stay in business. Providers will ask you for your insurance information within the first few moments of meeting you, as they know what protocols they must follow depending on the insurance coverage you have. As a consumer of such services, you should have a very good understanding of how those business entities function. This is the beginning of providing an insider perspective, which seeks to give an understanding for why things might be done a certain way. Having understanding makes empathy and advocacy possible.

A not so fun fact: your insurance coverage changes within different healthcare settings. In 2023 the healthcare setting where you physically go to seek services plays a big part in defining your health plan coverage. At the same time, changes in the healthcare system are making it possible to receive hospital level services literally in your home. This book won't cover this in detail, the changes are starting small. The tip here is to ASK! Every time you or your loved one enter a healthcare setting you MUST flip over your insurance card, call the customer service number, and ask about coverage and any changes in coverage which may have occurred since you subscribed to the policy. When you speak to your health insurance company, explain where you are using the name of the hospital, or emergency department, or even urgent care clinic. Ask them what services might not be covered, and what portion of the services they do cover you might be responsible for.

Understand who is "giving the orders" for services to be provided. In every healthcare setting there will be a physician whose credentials have been verified by that healthcare provider, giving them what we call "privileges to treat patients". As aforementioned, nothing can be done to you without the order coming from a physician or physician's assistant or a nurse practitioner. While it may not seem that the doctor is actually giving all of the orders in the moment, even in an emergency situation all of the actions taken are coming from doctor instructions. The emergency medical staff follow protocols which have been reviewed and authorized by medical directors. This is an important knowledge check. In western medicine, many administrative systems revolve around a simple concept of checking with the doctor and getting an order from that doctor to provide a treatment or service to you, which sometimes seems very logical to everyone and the time. To family members waiting for the doctor to call back and approve a simple pain medication for your loved one, the effort involved in obtaining that order feels burdensome.

Become a professional information gatherer! Asking questions which assist in information gathering is essential! This act of asking questions and gathering information makes it clear to everyone you are taking charge of your care and your goals. No matter which healthcare setting you or your loved one enters into, you are going to become an excellent and curious person who asks questions every day in order to obtain or confirm information driving the goals of care. Asking questions every day when you are not physically in the building brings on a new set of challenges. You begin a great game of phone tag. You may feel frustrated when you consistently leave messages, miss return phone calls, or don't get a timely call back. *Asking about electronic access to the data in the medical record in every care setting should be a top priority.* If you have access to the data, you can find answers to your questions. Technology is rapidly changing and more access to information is happening. Adoption of simple and easy to use technology will take time and vary within urban and rural markets. The message here is to *ask each provider if they have a portal where you or your loved one can have access to your electronic medical record* for when you are being cared for inside an institution. There are family portals available for both hospitals and skilled nursing facilities at the time of print- so ask as more are developed every day!

Who is in Charge of Your Care in an Institution?

Do you know who is calling the shots? Pardon the pun here, but it's imperative that you know how the healthcare system is designed and how it functions. The medical staff from whom you seek services are not always able to communicate with one another except in the forms of notes we call visit summaries. The moment you leave home in an emergency your primary care doctor will NOT be in charge of your care. Communication between your primary care doctor and every other doctor you see along the way will be limited to what they read in each other's documentation. By reading this section you will come to understand the name given to doctors in different care settings. Doctors who work inside hospital institutions are called "hospitalists" those who work inside a skilled nursing facility known as "SNFists". These doctors, and their associates care for you while you are in the emergency room, a hospital, acute rehabilitation, or a skilled nursing setting.

When you or a loved one enter into the US healthcare system in an urgent situation, the door to that system is an emergency department or the emergency room. During the registration process they will inquire as to who your primary care physician is. From this moment on, this doctor whom you have trusted and have confidence in is not going to be directing your care. The doctors in the emergency department are there to figure out what has changed in your health status and help formulate a plan for treatment, which may include admission to the hospital. While in the hospital, your primary care doctor will not be directing care for you. Depending on the problem, you will be referred to specialists in respective departments, like cardiology or orthopedics. You might see this specialist in the morning when they make rounds, but the rest of the time there is a hospitalist who is a general doctor or resident doctor who is responding to questions and calls from the nursing staff and will be coordinating a plan of care for you or your loved one.

You have to understand how the system is designed and how it functions in order to remain in control of that system. As a member who comes to seek treatment or care within the healthcare system, I really like to say that as individuals we make the decisions. The data needed to make those decisions is collected from the experts. And while I think this very academic approach is the best one to take for all of us, it's often not what actually occurs when you get into the healthcare system. The job for the advocate begins here. These physicians do not know you or your loved one's history. They practice medicine according to their formal training and practice experience which may not be what's best for you or your loved one.

Something you may not know about hospitals and nursing homes is that medical doctors or ancillary staff that work alongside a medical doctor like a nurse practitioner or a physician extender give instructions in the form of a doctor's order which are carried out by licensed nurses, therapists, and social workers. The person you may see come to the bedside most often could be a certified nursing assistant. All the treatment from the simple order needed for a special diet to the more complex orders needed for medications, laboratory testing, and activity and movement are given by the doctor. The moment you arrive in the healthcare system, the center of control changes from yourself or your loved one to the physician. The physician gives the orders, and all of these care workers provide care for you and must follow the physician's orders. I point this out as it is the first step in understanding how to successfully advocate for yourself or your loved one as you move into this system.

After 20 years of an active nursing career, my patient advocacy role was put to the ultimate test in 2009. In January 2009 my mother entered the healthcare system and spent four months in five different healthcare institutions, nine different rooms, and had 14 hospitalists in the last four months of her life. The number of times she actually met eye-to-eye with her primary oncologist was ZERO. The complexity of her case and ultimate demise was difficult enough. Explaining her history to each new hospitalist, emergency room doctor, and covering nurse was nearly impossible. My goal in sharing these stories is to offer practical strategies, questionnaires, and tips to navigate and advocate in the current model of care- that of being a hospitalist.

I've again learned this lesson through personal experience in advocating and helping my mother navigate through the healthcare system. My first tip is to be systematic in asking for data. Ask every day for a list of current orders - this can go beyond medications and include diet, activity, and testing. While it may seem simple, it's actually not that easy to obtain this information from very busy healthcare workers every single day. But I'm here to tell you that you have to ask these questions every single day in order to be fully informed, in complete control of healthcare decisions, and advocate for yourself or your loved one. This is especially true for any time of transition from one location of care to another. The number of errors that are made in the documentation between two healthcare settings is staggering. A simple omission of one medication and failing to have it written down on the continuity of care document will result in that drug not being ordered.

Some medications are not safe to stop abruptly, so an omission in some cases can create medical emergencies. While no one ever wants to make a mistake, the truth is mistakes happen. A big part of the emotions we feel comes from the belief we have that when you go into the healthcare system mistakes won't happen. The reality is they do, *and part of your job as an advocate is to ask questions and function in a way that those mistakes will be reduced.*

Tips for Transitioning From Home to the Hospital

- Always keep an updated list of your medications on hand for each medication - you should know the name (which could be either the brand name or the generic name) of the drug.
- For each medication you should know the dose amount that you actually take each day for each medication. If you take a different amount in the morning than you do at night, write these down.
- For each medication you should indicate how you get the drug into your body. This could be through your mouth, through your nose as an aerosol, on your skin as an ointment, in your eye as an ointment, etc. Medications are given through lots of different routes and it's important that you note the route which you take your medication.
- Keep a copy of your current health insurance card and identification card in your wallet. You can also make photocopies of these cards and keep the copies on your refrigerator in the event of an emergency.
- Keep a record of your primary care doctor's name, address, phone number, and fax number both in your wallet and on your refrigerator as a separate copy.
- Know your login to your online eHealth chart if you have one.

If you have an online my chart medical record portal, write down your username and password and give it to a member of your family whom you trust with your protected health information and would be willing to allow them to log in in your absence. It's often helpful for care providers who do not know you to look at your online records for most recent notes from your provider as well as testing and laboratory results. If you are willing to have a family member log in, they may be able to answer questions that the doctor has which might spare you unnecessary and additional testing.

Heading to the Emergency Department. What's Next?

Getting Registered and Sharing Insurance Information

When you first arrive in the emergency department either you or your loved one will need to present insurance and identification cards. It may seem odd to begin this section talking about payment for your care. Healthcare is a business. The more you put yourself in the shoes of a healthcare provider, and understand what drives the decisions made, the better you can navigate your own course. Let me also say that anyone can seek treatment for serious health issues in an emergency department in the US. The United States and other nations have passed laws requiring emergency rooms to treat all patients regardless of ability to pay. However, the majority of people seeking emergency care have an insurance provider who will pay a portion of the bill.

Let me ask you, do you know who will be paying the bill for the care you need? This may not be the first question on your mind after suffering an accident, illness, or change in health condition. It is however one of the first questions the institution you have entered would like answered. We are robotically trained to carry our identification cards and insurance cards and we dutifully present them during the registration process. While that feels like a warm and fuzzy getting to know you moment, it is in fact the institution determining who will primarily pay your bill. They will also determine if you have any supplemental insurance that will pay any balance left over, after your primary insurance has been processed. These are called your primary and secondary payers. There may or may not be some portion of the bill that you will be responsible for after all the bills have been processed.

You might be thinking, why does it matter who is paying the bill? Knowing who is responsible for payment impacts the decisions that are made and the actions taken. Let me give you a simple example. If you know you must pay a 50-dollar copayment before going to the emergency room, and you have a mild cough on a Sunday afternoon, you might ask yourself if you are truly "50 dollars" sick. You might decide to wait and call your primary care doctor for an appointment on Monday. This is a simple example, and one I use a lot when I'm teaching people the importance of gathering information in the "I" step of B.I.T.C.H.

Stay with me as I explore some basic principles which illustrate why it's important to determine who is paying the bill before any services are rendered. When I teach this concept I like to use the analogy of going out to dinner. Imagine that you were going to go out for dinner with another couple. I'm guessing the conversation with you and your spouse might go something like this:

You: "Have we picked a restaurant?"

Spouse: "Yes, the french restaurant on Main Street."

You: "Oh I love that place,they make the best desserts. Do you know if we will be accepting one check and simply sharing the cost equally or do you think they will want separate checks?"

Spouse: "I don't really know them that well. I'm not sure if they will want drinks and apps as well as dessert. Maybe we should just plan to have separate checks."

If you don't know the couple and you're not sure whether or not they are the type to order drinks and enjoy appetizers in addition to dessert, you might want to determine ahead of time whether or not you'll have two separate checks so that you can *control some of the cost* of your meal simply by what you order. What you do know is that you'll be responsible for some part of the bill, and since you know in advance that you're responsible for some part of the bill, *you make cost conscious choices about what you choose* throughout the dining experience. Guess what? Your insurance company knows they are paying the bill and they make choices about what providers, vendors, and services you may choose throughout your healthcare experience. See why it is so important?

Healthcare providers are businesses, and they need to determine immediately who is paying for the services they provide to you or your loved one *before* they provide services to you. They need to know exactly what company and which middleman they will be sending the bill to for the services that they provide to the patients. There can also be more than one organization that is going to pay the bill. We refer to this as having multiple insurance payers where one is primary payer and the other secondary payer. You may also know this as a "gap" plan. Where your second insurance covers some of the "gap" left by the first insurance. Of course, many of you have acknowledged that if your health insurance will not cover a service the healthcare provider may be submitting a bill directly to you for full reimbursement. The skilled nursing home space, which is the typical location for rehabilitation and restorative services provided after a short hospitalization stay, is often paid by either traditional Medicare, Managed Medicare, and in some cases parts of this services are covered by Medicaid.

Determining who is primarily responsible to pay for the stay, as well as determining if there is a secondary insurance payer who will cover costs not paid by the primary payer, are important milestones for the organization to determine literally as you are walking through the door. Insurance cards are utilized to determine if you are eligible for certain services to be covered and verifications with insurance companies begin often before many services are provided at all.

Maybe you're asking yourself why in a book on tips and tricks for advocacy we are spending so much time with a question of who's paying the bill. It's important that you understand that the organization who is writing a check for the services with which you are about to receive, known as the payer, wants you to go home as quickly as possible where the cost of care is typically the lowest. Days spent in the hospital, especially in intensive care units or critical care units, are the most expensive costs for payers. Followed by acute rehabilitation, the least costs are incurred in skilled nursing facilities or when living at home while receiving outpatient services or even no services at all. We will cover more topics in the area of who's paying for services when we talk about transition after hospital stays into a post-acute care setting. Controlling the cost of care is as important to your health insurance company as getting well is to you.

> **Tip**: Always have a copy of your current insurance card, both front and back, with you or "on the fridge" ready to go. If you change insurance providers or change in the open enrollment period, and then get sick before your new card arrives, you need to tell all providers that you have a change in insurance coverage coming, and give them the name of the new company, even if you don't have your card yet.

Tips For Thriving in an Emergency Department and Questions to Ask as You Prepare to Go Back "Home"

When you are evaluated in an emergency department, the team there needs to determine the next best place for you to receive ongoing care for whatever was ailing you in the "Oh Sh*t" moment.

The goal of the emergency department is to rapidly identify what's causing the change in your health status and explain to you what that usual health illness trajectory looks like, including possible complications and recovery time. There is a need to make a determination if you are able to go back home with supportive services or if you will require an inpatient hospital stay. This determination is a decision made by you or your loved one, given the data from the team in the emergency department. They will make a recommendation to you, and you ultimately have the final say in what you want to do.

Typically, these options include going back to your prior home, being admitted to the appropriate unit within a hospital, including an acute psychiatric hospital, or being discharged to a skilled nursing facility (SNF) for a short period of time. There are other options, and each case is unique, so if you don't see one of the typical options listed here you should ask to talk to the discharge planner in the emergency department about you or your loved one's unique needs.

Leaving against medical advice is never something I recommend people do. This book is all about advocacy and tips to be an informed consumer of the healthcare services available to you to reach your healthcare goals. There are times where the circumstances and situations may result in the medical team making a recommendation that you simply don't agree with at the moment. It is my experience that healthcare providers are willing to compromise when they can make compromises that do not severely put your health and safety at risk. Signing yourself out of an emergency department or a healthcare setting against medical advice, which is a technical status and includes a physical form that you will have to sign, is never suggested. When you make the declaration that you are willing to leave the healthcare setting against the medical advice that you have received, you are really going on your own from both a follow-up perspective as well as from an insurance perspective. What I have observed in these situations is that the person may not fully understand the information that's being communicated to them from the healthcare providers or feel a sense of urgency to get back home for a personal reason that the healthcare providers are not aware of. If you find yourself in this situation where you or someone you love is wanting to expedite removing themselves from a healthcare setting and is willing to do so by signing out against the advice of the medical team, it would be best to seek the advice of the discharge planner or social worker and consider alternatives.

Tips for Thriving in the ED:

- Bring your id and insurance card, your medication list, list of surgeries and conditions, activities of daily living, and advance directives – these should all be hanging on your refrigerator or hung on the back of the door to your apartment in a folder.
- Bring a cell phone and charger – you would be surprised how long you might be waiting and will want to connect with others.
- Be patient – LONG wait times in the emergency department are common.
- Ask if there is an opportunity for you or your loved one to log into the electronic medical record and have continuous access to the information that you need to guide your care goals for a loved one.
- Ask about the tests that were completed and what the results mean.
- Review the discharge instructions which they will print out for you and take a close look at any new medications they are prescribing.
- Ask if the new medications take the place of any of your old (from the fridge list) medications. In other words, do you

---

> stop one of your old medications while taking the new medication?
>
> - They will tell you to follow up with your primary care doctor- be sure to call them on the next business day and make an appointment.

For some of you your trip to the emergency department will result in an admission into the hospital. Depending upon your specific clinical needs, you will be admitted into an appropriate department to receive those services. For example, a problem with your heart will lead to you being admitted into the cardiology services and, depending upon the seriousness of your condition, you will be placed in an appropriate level of intensity for receiving those services. If you need very frequent monitoring and adjustments in medications, you may be placed in the intensive care unit where typically the nurse caring for you will be taking care of you and one or two other people. If your condition requires less frequent monitoring, you will be admitted to one of the general floors of the hospital where the nurse caring for you may have anywhere from 8-10 other people to take care of. When you are asking yourself "where's my nurse?" keep in mind the floor you are on, and the nurse-to-patient ratios, meaning that the nurse is providing care and sharing their time with you and other people. Time is limited. A nurse with 10 patients working a 12-hour shift can have no more than 72 total minutes to dedicate to any of your care needs. If you do the math you will realize 72 minutes assumes no break and no lunch for the nurse which is common. Regardless of what floor you are on in a hospital, the following section will help you or your loved one navigate and advocate for your care needs.

Thriving in an Acute Hospital setting; Daily Questions to Ask when You are in a Hospital

For those requiring an inpatient hospital stay, you will want to know if you are being admitted or simply observed. This is often a point of confusion for any of us since when we leave the emergency department and "go upstairs" or "get a room" we think that we are admitted to the hospital as an inpatient of that facility. Access to additional supportive services through Traditional Medicare insurance requires a three-night inpatient stay in a hospital setting. This three-day requirement has been waived by many managed care insurance providers for Managed Medicare, and during the COVID pandemic in 2021 was waived for Traditional Medicare beneficiaries as well. In the absence of the three-night stay minimum, or inpatient admission status in a hospital, access to a skilled nursing facility for rehabilitation services before going home would not be covered by Traditional Medicare. If you or your loved one are in the hospital and you are focused on understanding the new change in your health condition and the recommended treatments and services, chances are you're not thinking about the technical nature of your inpatient stay. That's another reason why this book is an essential read for you. Asking the right questions can ensure that you know if your inpatient stay has started, and you should also know that in order to access your Medicare benefits you're going to stay in that hospital for at least three overnights as the official attendance is taken each day at midnight in the US healthcare system. There will be a case manager or social worker at the hospital that can help you in getting an answer to this question. He or she also knows this information, as does the institution, but this book isn't about what healthcare providers know; this book is about how you should educate yourself and advocate for yourself or a loved one to ensure success as you move through the healthcare system. So ask the question of *if you are being admitted to the hospital or if you are in a status called "observation"* in the hospital. If there is any uncertainty in your mind about who your insurance provider is, go back to that section of the book on who's paying the bill and review.

When you or someone you love is in the hospital, staying on top of changes in the plan of care every day is the focus for the advocate. In this section I'll review some tips and strategies that, when you follow every day, make surviving and thriving more plausible. These steps should be taken in order they are presented, and I realize step one might be a doozie.

1. Determine one member of your family to be the key contact with the care provider
2. Ask the care provider if there is a family portal where you can see details of the care provided
3. Ask for the phone number, name and role of the one person you can call with questions
4. Create a group text message in your phone where you will text updates
5. Ask for a list of medication, diet, treatment, and testing orders *every day*

Did I really just say ask for a list of medications every day? Yes, that is my professional and personal advice from experiences I went through as an advocate. Here is how I approach that technique with the care team. I introduce myself and assure them that I know how busy they are, and I thank them in advance for caring for my loved one. Then I ask if they have any family portals where I can see how my loved one's day has been, including the medications they took that day. I communicate openly my intention to check these details every day. If no portal exists, I ask for the best phone number and time of day that I can call and speak with a staff person to get these answers. I reassure them that I am the point person for the family, and family updates will come from me. Then I tell them I have a paper and pen and I am ready for the medication list.

Recall that this book opened up with the reminder that the human body is a very large chemistry lab, and with that image in mind you can understand why consistently asking about medications is a top priority. Communicate this request clearly and simply to the caregivers in the system where you are. Technology is rapidly changing access to information for patients and family. The 21st Century Cures Act is a federal regulation that actually sets a rule that patients and their families have access to all medical record information upon request in a timely fashion. As a result of technology systems improving, you can see in near real time the order for yourself or your loved one. *Ask about this.* You may find that there is an online web portal like a My E-chart where you or your loved one can be accessing key information. You may find that there is a family portal application that not only allows access to the information, but also supports communication between yourself and the caregivers for your loved one. Technology solutions that facilitate family and provider communications make it easier for information to be exchanged, and less errors occur due to miscommunication.

I could share a handful of stories with you through the years of family and friends who have come to me for advice while a loved one was moving through the healthcare system. Often times medications are changed, and the family or patient has no idea of how things have been ordered or why. I don't mean to share this in a judgmental way of the people who are providing care; in fact, the caregivers are overburdened and stretched very thin every day. Remaining grateful for the time and attention that they give to your loved one or to yourself is essential. However grateful, you can never let your guard down to not ask and advocate for yourself or your loved one. In times when I failed to do this myself, well-meaning hospitalist staff would change medications, drug classifications, or the time of day that medications were ordered all in an effort to improve a loved one's health status. However, not knowing the history in many cases meant these changes had poor health and quality of life results. When this happened to my mother, I was traveling for work and missed calling one day. I returned 3 days later to find my mother had gained 15 pounds of fluid weight. The well intentioned hospitalist had changed her "pee pill" from her usual dose and time of day to a routine more aligned with the newer research. What they did not know is that my mother had failed on this routine before. They did not ask her or me, and I had failed to make my daily calls. This is why I have learned how important it is to ask every day for updates. Furthermore, the changes which occurred without review with my mom or myself were incredibly annoying. When I called every day, I took control like the "T" in B.I.T.C.H and I was less irritated when I did learn of changes that were being made, and I could ask for an explanation why. The care teams learn quickly that I am going to call, and they start calling me *before* changes are made.

Through these experiences I learned that I must ask these questions every single day that someone I love is in an institutional care setting. Gather your family and agree on one person to contact and communicate with the care provider's main contact. Identifying one key contact member in your family to communicate with the healthcare setting makes care coordination effective and efficient for the healthcare providers. Expect some delays and the emotion which comes with waiting. Frustration may emerge even when you feel you have mastered the contents of this book. I recently had a personal experience where my family member was in the hospital with COVID. I was reminded of all of the advice that I have been writing in this book and needed to put my own advice into action. One perspective I had forgotten about was preparing to be frustrated. Even when you do all the right things and you ask all the right questions, you will not always get a timely response, and you may not even get the outcome from the healthcare setting that you desired. These emotions are intense and can be consuming if you don't watch out for them.

Let's talk through a couple of examples. In this book I remind you that there are going to be a lot of questions asked, especially around medications. To start, when the phone rang at 7:00AM the morning of the first day after admission, I was not surprised that the nurses asked me to complete a medication reconciliation review. She listed the exact medications I knew my loved one was taking. I did not need to bother the nursing staff for another check-in that day. The following day I called and left a message. It took six hours for the nurses to get back to me, and when I did speak with the nurse and asked my routine question of reviewing current active medication orders, it was surprising that there was a prescription missing.

Clearly, the act of doing a medication reconciliation is to prevent medication errors, and I was questioning why a key medication used to thin the blood known as Coumadin was missing from my loved one's orders. I requested that the doctor give me a call to explain the rationale behind not using the medication assuming that it was an intentional decision and not a medication omission. I waited 24 hours and did not receive a phone call. I then placed another call and, while speaking with the nurse, learned that the medication order had been omitted in error.

At this point I was feeling exasperated and I was reminded that this is an important point to mention in this book. Even when you follow all of the right steps, you ask all the right questions, and you are your own B.I.T.C.H. advocate, you are still going to find mistakes made by the healthcare system. There will be emotions provoked. To be honest, those mistakes are the reason that these tips are written as suggestions and essential for you to follow. I know this sounds odd, but I am trying to replace negative emotions with positive ones, like a mini celebration that an error was caught! Had I not been consistently following my own advice; this medication error omission may have gone on for several more days with potentially terrible health outcomes for my loved one. I took a deep breath and told myself: *Follow the plan, ask the questions, gather the Information, communicate your concerns, and get back to coordinating the care you or your loved one needs for getting "home".*

These care providers were appreciative of my questioning and grateful that through review the omission was caught, and the medication was restarted. Let me assure you, as a nurse avoiding a mistake by any means is the goal. You might be wondering if all the questions you ask are going to upset the nurses. When I was working in rehabilitation, I remember the first time one of my patients asked me about a pill they did not recognize in the little white pill cup I handed them. I explained what the pill was, and what it was for. I was sure I had prepared them correctly. Then I paused and said I would double check and come right back. I had made a mistake in preparation of the medications. I was so very grateful that they had looked in the cup and asked me to double check them. I realized how helpful they had been to me! Your knowledge of what you should be taking, and your review of the medications are helpful to the nurse and impact the outcomes! *Care providers appreciate well intended advocates so keep it up.*

Ask to confirm your or your loved one's advance directives status. As I mentioned in an earlier chapter of this book, defining your advance directives is important for you to be able to make sure the caregivers know what instructions you want followed in the event of a change in health status. This is often difficult to communicate during the transition into an emergency department or hospital setting. Even when you do all the right things and bring your advance directives in your hand into a healthcare system, you may find that not every member of the team is equipped with the accurate advance care plan instructions which you have provided.

A recent example came from the same stay when my loved one was in the hospital with COVID. During the first day I had a conversation with the hospital staff, they asked me to confirm the code status of a "full code". A full code means in the event that one's heart stops beating, you want the care team to try everything to get it going again.

The opposite of this is an order "do not resuscitate" or DNR. I communicated that there was an advance directive in place and that the wish was for a "do not resuscitate order" to be on the chart. A physical copy of those instructions was provided later that same day to the hospital staff for entry into the chart. Upon review of the physician's notes the following day, I noted the physician indicated a full code status for my loved one. I brought this inconsistency/inaccuracy to the attention of the facility, and at that time they were unable to find the physical hard copy which had been provided the day before of the advance directives. We were then provided with a blank form to complete the advance directives for this institution, and while that form was filled out and awaiting signature of the patient, the healthcare record continued to list my loved one as a full code. 24 hours later while reviewing the medical record for a completely different reason, the omitted medication of Coumadin, I noticed the physician note still had my loved one listed as a "full code". In the first part of this book we talked about completing advance directives. My loved one had done their job, and even took the copy from the refrigerator to the hospital with them, and still due to some error, the record did not reflect their wishes. Just another example of how even though you are doing the right advocacy work, it may take more than one or two communication events to clearly and completely express the desires and care needs of your loved one. Consistency is important and will get the results necessary.

Frustration is an emotion that I was experiencing that week, saying to myself "I can't even make this stuff up". This was a stark reminder of how important it was that I focused on completing this work, and that you finish reading this book and that you reread it each time you have a loved one in a healthcare setting. If you have a person to look after, it's imperative you have some strategies for doing that job well!

The healthcare staff team, made up of mostly doctors and nurses, are doing amazing work and as consumers of their caregiving skills, we all need to recognize them! None of them come to work expecting to make a mistake. My observation is that the staff have so many people assigned to them during a shift that they are not capable of tending to all of the details accurately. Your job as an advocate is to keep track of only one loved one at a time, and therefore your job is to call and ask questions as many times as is necessary to get the desired healthcare result. I'm happy to say that my loved one was able to go home and did not have any complications from the medication omission, did not have any complications from the inaccurate code status, and was able to return home safely. These kinds of mistakes take place every day and *it's advocates like you and I who make a difference in the outcomes* of the care. Stay vigilant even when it feels daunting.

Once you or your loved one have been stabilized in the hospital, the case manager or social worker will immediately begin talking with you about leaving the hospital. Sometimes this feels really fast - this almost always feels really fast. Keep a few things in mind: to be very honest the one place you never want to be is in the hospital. Maybe this sounds completely logical to you, but the reason I'm saying this is that in the hospital setting you're not able to follow your normal routine, the one that you described just a few pages ago.

Our bodies are little systems and they do better when we function in a consistent way every day. When you enter the hospital it becomes very irregular if you're lying in bed for hours. You may not be getting up alone, as you are not in your normal setting and may not have the right equipment. You are not having your regular meals; your routines and sense of balance are off to your body. Most of us want to get out of the hospital as quickly as possible and take a step closer to home, to where our normal balance and our normal flow for our body is established.

Your insurance company also wants you to get out of the hospital as quickly as possible since this is the most expensive care center and they are paying your bill. They would very much like you to move to a lower cost care center. This may sound funny or snarky, and I'm not saying they don't care about the outcomes of your health, because they do. What I am saying is that they are in business to minimize the cost of care at the same time as providing high quality and high satisfaction to you as a consumer of their services.

So again, once you've barely settled into the hospital someone's going to be talking to you about getting out. For many people there will be a need for a little more time for rehabilitation and recuperating before going back home. Preparing for that transition to a skilled nursing facility is what we're going to cover next. It's an important decision about where you go and one that shouldn't just be made on a limited set of data, so let's talk about the data elements that you should use to consider where you might go.

Leaving the Hospital for a Care Setting Other than "Home": Avoiding the Transitional "Gaps"

As you or your loved one stabilize your condition in the hospital, determining the next less costly sight of care for you to continue rehabilitation will be determined. As I mentioned, the health insurance plan or the payer who is writing a check for your care would very much like you to move as quickly as possible from the higher cost settings to lower cost settings. Hospitals per day price is much more expensive than the cost of care per day in a skilled nursing facility. Depending upon the services that you need, you may not even need to go to a skilled nursing facility for a short stay rehab course - you may find that you're able to go directly home with services in your home. In many instances after an acute illness which results in a hospitalization, a short course of inpatient rehabilitation at a skilled nursing facility may be recommended.

As you prepare to leave the hospital and enter any other care setting which might include either a skilled nursing rehabilitation or acute rehabilitation setting, recognize that this transition makes you vulnerable to information sharing. This should be accurate and complete between the two healthcare providers, however, is often fraught with error. Information and Communication, the "I" and "C" in B.I.T.C.H., are the central characters of this chapter.

One or two days before you leave the hospital you should ask for a complete list of your current medication orders, including the current order for your diet, activity, and weight bearing status if you've had any orthopedic conditions. The hospital will provide a continuity of care document to the post-acute provider who will be caring for you next. While it seems that all the information is accurate, often there are omissions and gaps.

As an advocate you are going to want to ask a lot of questions in preparation for transition. After reviewing the list of medications that you or your loved one are taking one to two days prior to discharge, you should ask if every one of those medications is going to be available to you in the way or the route with which you've been receiving them at your next provider location.

Not all skilled nursing facilities provide the same degree of intensive clinical interventions. If you have been requiring an intravenous for pain medication, hydration, or antibiotics you may find that at the skilled nursing facility those problems are going to be addressed using medications that you can take by mouth instead of medications that are delivered through intravenous. These changes in medication planning often have an impact on the quality of the transfer and the comfort of your loved one.

Pain management is one area in particular where transitions can be incredibly challenging for the patient. This can be especially true for a patient who was transitioning from IV pain medication to oral pain medication as is often the case since this transition tends to happen at the same time you are discharged from the hospital and admitted into the skilled nursing facility. Since the admission process including transportation can take several hours, patients are often left with inadequate medication for pain management. Imagine going through the fear and anxiety of transitioning to a skilled nursing facility for rehabilitation, coupled with increase in pain, which may result in excruciating pain as the hours wear on, and no medication is forthcoming. The skilled nursing facility has to first receive the written copy of the orders, then verify those copied orders with the physician who will be providing care and overseeing your loved one's care in the skilled nursing facility. Those conversations can often take hours, leaving your loved one with no ordered pain medication and therefore no pain relief.

You might be thinking that the doctor who was writing the orders at the hospital would also be authorizing those same orders inside the skilled nursing facility; however, this is not the case. As I mentioned in Chapter One, each institution has physicians on staff who are credentialed and able to write orders for patients who are receiving care in those facilities. Because of this, the physician in the hospital who has been caring for your loved one for a period of time is not the physician who's going to continue to order medications for your loved one in the skilled nursing facility or the acute rehab facility.

We are sending information from one care team to another and, frankly, doctors don't all have the same opinions on how to tackle certain problems. This is how your loved one ends up with sudden changes in the plan of care based on the opinion of the physicians supervising that care. Again, this is the perfect role for an advocate. When you have taken the time to figure out what best works for yourself or your loved one continuing on the example of pain management, the last thing you want is the opinion of a different physician to change that plan, especially when things are going really well. So this is a time for you, as a patient, to advocate, or if you're advocating for a loved one to speak up and ask in advance if all of the medications that the hospital physician currently has on order are going to be available in the exact form at the skilled nursing facility.

If they're not going to be available in the exact same form, then you need to ask what medications the doctor plans to change you or your loved one onto and request that that change be made prior to discharge from the hospital. It's better to try a new medication and make sure that you get effective pain relief without any allergic reaction in the hospital before transferring to a skilled nursing facility and having those first one or two days be filled with excruciating pain. Often times patients who suffer this kind of pain upon transition will be sent back to the hospital for further pain management evaluation when in fact this evaluation could have taken place prior to the transition. These are the kinds of complications and costly experiments which can be avoided with good advocacy.

What if You or Your Loved One *Do Not WANT* to Go to "Rehab"?

Understand that your physical limitations or those of your loved one will not magically improve when you pull into your home driveway. Often, upon leaving the hospital, patients believe that if they just get home into their own environment their physical limitations which may have been as a result of a sudden change in health status, a fall, or infection are going to magically disappear. I can assure you as a nurse, changes in health condition and decline in functional ability take time and effort to recover from.

Skilled nursing facilities serve an essential role in the healthcare continuum as short-term rehabilitation and recovery providers. The perception of SNFs is not what the media would have you think. The wide range of people who are served in care settings and the diversity of skills needed among the staff are impressive. This is the care setting where I have served in various roles for nearly 30 years. As of 2023, there are about 1.4 million residents in U.S. nursing homes. Thousands of Americans every year receive care at skilled nursing facilities as a short stay patient along the care continuum in the direction of home.

Only four percent of seniors in the United States live long term in nursing homes. This is a location where daily skilled services following a three-day hospital stay, can be provided for up to 100 days. Providing skilled services is required and the person receiving those services is making reasonable progress towards a prior level of function.

Okay so that was a very technical definition of a skilled nursing facility. Many of you think of a nursing home as a place to move your loved one to, out of their community when they require more help than can be provided in the home. In this scenario you might think they are going to live out the rest of their life in a nursing home. While most nursing homes provide both short stay (less than 100 days) and long stay (over 100 days), most facilities have separate units for these two groups. Those coming for a short course of rehabilitation with the goal of returning to home in most cases will be in a defined space with other short stay people. The image you might have in mind from the media is most likely not what you will see upon admission. Short stay rehabilitation units do a phenomenal job allowing people to recover from a change in health, regain strength and function, and give some time for healing. The professionals there are trained to monitor and stabilize a wide variety of acute health changes, assisting you as you strive to regain independence and return home.

A short stay in an acute rehab hospital, a skilled nursing facility, or in some instances an assisted living setting where the services of licensed nurses and licensed therapists are on site and available around the clock up to seven days per week may be needed for optimal recovery and successful discharge to home. Give yourself some space to accept this investment of time in your own healing process. As an advocate for your loved one, you may need to help them see that a short stay in a skilled nursing facility may be warranted. When I am helping family and friends to see this perspective, I begin by getting the patient to describe their prior level of function in detail. I have them tell me about each day, each morning how they go to the bathroom, how they get dressed, how they bathe, how they prepare meals, how they take food, and how they interact with the community. This prior level of function represents the independence that they had just before admission to the hospital. While most of us as humans want to go home as quickly as possible, I think what we really want is to regain our independence as much and as quickly as we can. Instead of thinking about going home in a finite number of days, they are thinking that going to a nursing home after the hospital might be considered undesirable. I always talk about the quality of their life and the independence that they had prior to their illness. I encourage them to evaluate honestly if they are currently at that same level of functional independence and quality of life as before. Then I remind them that these are benefits which they are entitled to for those who are covered under Medicare, Managed Medicare, or some might be duly eligible for Medicare and Medicaid insurance payments. This allows them to look at the time in the skilled nursing facility as investing their own time in the quality of their life and the independence which they wish to regain.

The first question you or your loved one are most likely going to ask, or be asked by family and friends, is how long will you or your loved one be in the skilled nursing rehab? The care team will give an estimate based on how much change in your condition has occurred with your recent change in health status. The way that you leverage your time in a skilled nursing facility is an investment that you make for yourself. The takeaway of this point is to rethink one's physical, mental, and clinical needs and not get caught up in thinking that a short stay at a nursing home is a bad thing. Now that you or your loved one sees the benefits from a short course of skilled rehabilitation, we will return to the job of advocating. Let's go!

Being Your Own Best Advocate

Over the past 30 plus years of working in this industry and helping family and friends move through a post-acute experience, I'm very surprised to see that the expectation is that the facility care providers will take a lead role in advocating and communicating the needs of the patient. As hard as that is to understand, I want you to remember that when one nurse comes into work at a nursing home he or she could be assigned anywhere from 10 to 30 patients depending upon the time of day that they are working and the overall acuity or illness level of those patients. That one human nurse cannot possibly think holistically and remember all of the data and details of your loved one. You need to assume the role of quarterback at this junction in time. What do I mean by using this analogy? You're the one who's going to have to rely on your knowledge of yourself or your loved one. Think of the work you did in the first part of this book, getting prepared and documenting advanced directives, usual routines, and medication rituals. You will need to take a leadership role, knowing yourself or advocating for your loved one. You will need to take time to talk to the facility staff, agree on a plan of care, and then be part of how that plan is executed. You will have the responsibility of staying on top of all of the details involved in your or your loved one's plan. There will be staff who will help partner with you, and they are incredible leaders in their organizations. They also have 10 to 30 other people like you to assist. Taking personal accountability for communication, collaboration, and coordination lets everyone on the care team know you are determined to get home.

As an advocate you are already prepared each day because you have asked for and received a list of what is currently ordered for medications, diet, and activity. As the quarterback, you're going to want to know what the general plan is each day and what the schedule is like in the institution. Of course, institutions have schedules in order to take care of the needs of many human beings for bathing, dressing, medication, etc. As such, institutional approaches to care have to be taken for efficiency. What that means is that in general all meals are served at the same time each day and in certain dining room locations.

Any special needs that you have for eating early or having a snack later can be met, but they have to be communicated and monitored by the quarterback. The nurse who comes on at three in the afternoon may not know that you had a late lunch, and you want a late dinner. For example, these are individual details that when communicated to the nurse are met with success. So that's what I mean when I say prepare to be the daily quarterback. It's a very important job but it's also a job that is tiring and I want to acknowledge that.

It's not to say that some things won't go right without you or a loved one acting as the quarterback. The care team of nurses, nursing assistants, therapists, social workers, and all of the staff who work in post-acute facilities know the plan for your care, they communicate to one another continuously, and are incredibly dedicated individuals. The sheer volume of patients to working people creates opportunities for small things to fall through the cracks. Like I said, if it's really important to you to have a late evening snack before bed and that helps you have a good night's sleep, then your advocate needs to emphasize the importance of that late night snack and make sure that they communicate it to the oncoming or the human person who actually shows up to work each and every day. You might be thinking, "It's the same nurse as last night. Why do I need to remind them?" In many instances it will be the same person multiple days in a row, and at some point you might feel like your constant questioning and reminding is an annoyance to them. I'm asking you to ignore those feelings and to just continue to ask the questions and state the important reminders. I have been in the shoes of those nurses. I assure you the care team will appreciate your advocacy "reminders", especially when you communicate your intentions to assist in making sure the needs of you or your loved one are met. Remember the goal is to thrive, not just survive this post-acute experience.

Choosing a Post-Acute Care Provider Considering the Location and Proximity to Your Home or Closest Visitor

It may seem obvious that you prefer to go to a skilled nursing facility for your rehab stay which is closest to your home, and this is a valid item for consideration; however, there are a couple of other data elements to think through. You may want to rehab in a facility which is closest to your advocate who is going to help you navigate through the following tips and suggestions from this book. You may also choose a rehab location that is close to your spouse if visiting you on a daily basis under normal circumstances is important to you and to them. For many, this represents the first time living separated for more than a few days and that separation can be quite difficult. A daily visit can help ease the mental and emotional transition of spending extensive time away from one another.

In addition to the physical location, you will want to consider the reputation of the facility that you are entering. Reputation is interesting. It can form from hearing stories of peers or friends who have gone through the rehab program at a location or it can form from stories in the media, which are often misrepresentative of the good care that is otherwise provided at that location. It can also be assessed online at carecompare.com using a Five-Star rating system which was designed with consumers in mind to give you information about skilled nursing facilities. One point I want to make is that unlike a Yelp review or other online review websites, consumers don't directly contribute to the Five-Star rating system. If you have a great experience at a skilled nursing facility you can send them a card, a letter, a basket of flowers, or maybe some candy. But you can't go online and write a review that gets considered and factored into the Five-Star rating score that you're going to see when you go to carecompare.com. The only consumer voice that is reflected in the Five-Star rating system would be the results of a complaint, which if made to the state ombudsman office is investigated. Should that investigation find noncompliance of care, it can reach the level of a citation and that complaint and situation would be expressed in the Five-Star rating system in the survey portion. What I'm saying here is that while there is some good information on carecompare.com, it's not going to tell you the whole story of the skilled nursing facility which you are about to enter.

When I do look at carecompare.com I look for staffing to be above average and for quality to be at or above average. Keeping in mind that the only professionals that count in the staffing are registered nurses, LPNs, and CNAs. There are a lot of professionals working in the SNF that are not shown in those numbers today. For example, the skilled PT, OT, and SLP therapy team members which would provide your rehab program directly to you are not included in those staffing numbers nor anywhere in the Five-Star rating. However, the quality of those departments and the programs offered usually have a known reputation and it helps to ask for feedback from your physician and any of your family or friends who may have received their rehabilitation at that same location.

Still in the Hospital ...BUT Planning a Move to a Rehab or a Skilled Nursing Facility

Think of this section the way you might get ready for an upcoming trip. You have not left yet, but you are planning ahead, making a packing list, imagining what you might need when you arrive, or trying to figure out what you might forget. Only in this case you are going to leverage my expertise and learn from my experiences, so you show up with everything you need, and there are less surprises.

Even before you arrive at the rehab facility you're going to need to bring your own B.I.T.C.H. into the conversation. Once you have chosen a location for your rehabilitation and they have been able to offer you a bed for admission, you should begin to think about getting home. Even before you have left the hospital, start thinking about what you're going to need to be able to do for yourself or what your loved one will be able to do for themselves, in order to *safely return home and stay home.*

I know that sounds like an obvious statement, however, in the United States many people who enter the hospital find themselves returning to the hospital within 30 days of a discharge. This is a statistic and outcome of care that is a priority of focus in the US healthcare system. Think of it like a 30-day warranty on a product that you purchase. If you invest thousands of dollars in a new appliance you certainly don't want to have any problems with it in the first 30 days, and that seems like a minimum to me. So there is this balancing act between moving quickly from an expensive care setting like the hospital to a skilled rehab facility or skilled nursing facility and the intense urgency we all feel to get back home. When balancing that urge to get back home with the medical stability that is needed to STAY at home, a 30-day warranty is what we are striving to achieve. Going back home too quickly may result in another hospitalization in those first 30 days.

The balance that we're looking for is making sure that when you do get back home you have the skills, knowledge, and physical capability of being cared for safely in your home. The ultimate goal is not returning to the hospital - certainly not in the first 30 days after discharge. I mention this concept so that you can be thinking about this balance as well. Being aware of the momentum in the healthcare system is part of being informed, and it's how you advocate for yourself while having empathy and an understanding of the objectives they're trying to achieve within their business organization.

Even before you leave the hospital you should begin to think about those activities of daily living, your usual abilities to care for yourself, and what you're capable of doing today and thinking about the distance or the difference between those two. This is where you want to take a look back over your usual activities of daily living that you documented and left on your refrigerator. Ask yourself, are you functioning at this level today? Are you honestly ready to return to home and do all of those activities at the same prior level of function with both strength, endurance, and confidence? If the answer is no, you would most likely benefit from a short stay in a rehab or skilled nursing facility to achieve that prior level of function. There is no magic carpet that is going to fly you home and return you to your prior level of function. You are going to have to work hard to achieve that at the rehab facility.

Here is a list of questions you should ask and get the answer to before transitioning to a short-term rehabilitation center:

- What skilled services will I have? Physical therapy? Occupational therapy? Speech therapy? Nursing?
- How many hours per day, and days of the week will these skilled services be provided to me?
- Do I have any weight bearing restrictions or any movement restrictions as a result of my condition that my therapy team will need to know about?
- When, in terms of weeks, or by what date will the next diagnostic procedure be completed that would determine a change in those weight bearing or movement restrictions?
- What is the plan for pain management during the day of transition and after admission?
- Are there any services I am currently receiving that won't continue in the nursing home, examples IV medications for pain, IV antibiotics for infections? What is the plan for when these services change?
- What are your current dietary orders?

Preparing for the Transition to a Skilled Nursing Facility for Rehabilitation or an Acute Rehab Facility.

Knowing what to expect upon transition to a skilled nursing facility or an acute rehabilitation center can reduce your fear of the transition and improve the clarity and focus of your questions. The reason for asking questions is to gather information. Recall the B.I.T.C.H. framework, and prepare to ask lots of questions. If you are unsure what data you need, you don't know what questions to ask, right? This section will help you think through the data you need and the questions to ask. Getting to know the key players in that institution, their essential role, and how you can leverage the information, in order to communicate your goals and plans for getting back home are key. Later we will explore the titles of the people you will meet in a skilled nursing facility, and what they do to help you. This section will help you plan ahead and be ready for the next stop on your journey.

Prior to admission into a skilled nursing facility, the admission coordinator will verify with your insurance company that you have coverage to be treated in a skilled nursing facility for a short period of time. You may hear this explained to you if you have a Managed Medicare health plan as an initial authorization for coverage followed by a number of days which the insurance company has authorized that coverage.

Anytime you move from one care location to another you're going to experience what I call a "vulnerable transition". This is a time where your needs and your care team are about to change. This makes you as a patient very vulnerable as the possibility for lost information is real. This is a great time to ramp up your advocacy functions, asking lots of questions every single day about current orders, and asking questions before the transition occurs about the services and availability of the same services to be received in the nursing home. You or your family member may be the most up to date, and accurate source for all the medical information care providers need to know. Even though there are systems in place to transfer your details, sometimes details get missed, or the details change. Communication and care collaboration depend on your advocacy especially during a vulnerable transition. See the tips box for questions to ask.

There are oftentimes assumptions made that the care that you receive at the hospital will be the exact same care that you receive at a skilled nursing facility. In some instances those assumptions are very wrong. For example, if you're receiving pain management through IV medication in the hospital and you finally get to a place where you're quite comfortable and movement is eased by the pain medication, you may be surprised to learn that the nursing home where you have been planning to discharge does not offer IV pain medication administration. Oftentimes on the day of your transfer from the hospital to the skilled nursing facility the hospitalist will change the pain medication order from the IV drug to an oral drug. Those orders will be transferred to the skilled nursing facility, and this will be your new plan for managing your pain. Although this is a normal and usual approach to reducing pain medication, it is also an experiment since we don't really know how well that new oral pain medication is going to do at controlling your pain. Unfortunately for many, what happens is the transition to the skilled nursing facility fails as the patient arrives at the new location with new medication orders, oftentimes causing a delay in receiving their pain medication per the schedule. While waiting for the medication to arrive, the patient gets horrible or excruciating pain. None of us need to think for a minute about whether we would want to experience this kind of arrival at our new rehab center.

In fact, none of us want to experience horrible or excruciating pain even for 10 or 15 minutes, and oftentimes upon these transitions patients are waiting hours for appropriate medications to arrive from pharmacies. Then more time is spent waiting for staff to have time to administer the medication, and then you wait a little bit longer for the medication to begin to work before you can even evaluate if that medication is effective. Asking questions prior to transition around the plan for pain management is one example, but I'm really talking about all order management being an essential job for the caregiver advocate prior to any transition. Some questions to ask yourself are what were any recent problems in the hospital which are now under control, and do you know how that control was achieved? For this example with pain, do I know how the pain was managed? If it's a question about medical management of other conditions, are you informed of the current diet, medication, and activity orders which came together to control or bring some balance back to that health condition? These are the kinds of questions that you want to ask to the care coordinator at the hospital, who is also coordinating the transfer to the skilled nursing facility.

Another important question to ask is around any physical mobility restrictions that you may have. This will also include the amount of weight that you are able to bear on any of your arms and legs. Oftentimes after having an orthopedic injury there is a restriction referred to as a "weight bearing status" which is given by the orthopedic doctor in the form of a physical order. This weight bearing status will determine what the physical therapist and occupational therapist must follow for restrictions while working with you in your rehab stay. Your insurance company will be interested in knowing what the weight bearing status restrictions are for you as they know that when you are non-weight bearing there are limitations to what the therapy team can do with you. This may impact the amount of time that they are willing to authorize inpatient rehabilitation for. Armed with information and ready to communicate those details, you are now an informed consumer ready to take control of our health outcomes and rock through rehabilitation so you can get back home.

If you are in need of more than three hours of skilled therapy services each day, you might be referred to an acute rehabilitation hospital where you can also receive the same skilled services at a more intense level. This is less common but can occur as a discharge from the hospital to an acute rehabilitation hospital or care center. The tips for transitioning from one care provider to another remain the same no matter which level of service you're going to receive. Focusing on medications, activities, restrictions on movement or weight bearing, the need for routine or follow up laboratory testing, dietary restrictions, and of course your most current advance directive are essential documents that you want to have mastery of during the time of transition.

Getting to Know the Professionals Who Specialize in Skilled Nursing and Rehabilitation Facilities

Welcome to rehabilitation! There is a whole new cast of professionals that you will leverage to get yourself back home. In this section I will introduce you to some very important people, their roles, and common titles. Knowing who does what and what they are called is an important piece of information that you will need to feel less like an impostor in this new environment, and more in control of advocating for your own care needs.

The leadership in a skilled nursing facility consists traditionally of two main leaders: the administrator, who is a licensed member of the team and is the leader of the organization, and the director of nurses, who is a licensed, registered nurse and is the leader of the clinical services provided.

Together these two human beings run the business at that one local facility. If the skilled nursing facility is owned by a larger parent corporation, there may also be regional or corporate staff who oversee multiple buildings. Typically, you will interact with the staff from this one facility. You may have met the admissions coordinator, sometimes referred to as a hospital liaison, while you were in the hospital. These are staff who work for the nursing home and meet patients in the hospital. They work to understand the needs that you have for recovery and explain to you the services provided in the nursing home which can meet those recovery needs.

Once you have arrived at the skilled nursing facility one of the first faces that you will see is your admissions coordinator who will come to your room to greet you and welcome you. After that, it will feel like a flurry of professionals are clamoring to get into your room and make their introductions and begin their professional assessment of you to form a plan for your care needs. In the skilled nursing facility you will have care provided to you by a licensed nurse who could be a registered nurse or a licensed practical nurse. There will be lots of certified nursing assistants. There will be licensed physical therapists, occupational therapists, and speech therapists, and depending upon what your recovery plan requires, one or all of these people will be introducing themselves to you within a few hours of your arrival at the nursing home. This may happen the next day if you arrive later in the evening. In addition to that care team, you will also have a case manager or a social worker who serves as an internal coordinator for the nursing home facility team and will do communications when required throughout your stay to your health insurance case manager.

It's important to know who the key players are in a skilled nursing facility and what role they will play in assisting you or your loved one to regain health and return home. If you noticed, I didn't mention your primary care doctor; remember your primary care doctor is not going to come and see you in most cases at a nursing home. In fact, the nursing home will have either a medical director or a handful of attending physicians, physician assistants, or nurse practitioners who frequent the facility, visiting new admissions and providing ongoing medical service care only during the course of your skilled nursing facility stay. Upon your discharge they will release your care back to your primary care doctor if you are returning home to the community.

Oftentimes this is the one person that you actually want to see on a daily basis, however in most cases you will not. The SNF doctors might come in and talk to the nurses about your care, and make changes, and may or may not see you each time. Patients and families have a hard time and can feel frustrated when most of the questions they ask around changes in service or patient's condition will be met with a response that includes communication to the doctor, and the nurse will acknowledge that he or she will not have an answer for you until they communicate and hear back from the doctor.

This is a common theme in all nursing homes across the country with patients because the physician really gives the orders, and no changes in care can be made without a physician's order. Recall from the earlier sections on this topic, the need for an order creates a bit of a bottleneck in getting change accomplished. Having some empathy for these humans who do super important jobs is an important goal of introducing you to them by role.

In the Beginning the Admission Coordinator or Liaison

Before you leave the hospital, you will have probably been talking with an admission liaison or admission coordinator. They are selling you a short course of inpatient rehabilitation services, and they are going to communicate your needs to the care team at the rehabilitation setting. Once you enter the skilled nursing facility this person will often come and say hello, typically on the day you arrive and may even require you to sign several documents required for admission. You can have these documents signed electronically in advance, or completed by a designated responsible party who may also be serving as your advocate. After you have done the admission paperwork you're probably not going to see this person again.

Case Managers or Social Workers, and Sometimes You Get Both!

Everyone who is admitted to a skilled nursing facility will have a case manager or a social worker who will help to coordinate the discharge plan for you. I know you've just barely arrived in the building and it seems a little strange to be thinking about leaving already, but as I mentioned in the previous chapter, everyone in the healthcare system, from the moment you enter, is thinking of how quickly they can stabilize you and prepare to discharge you home. Getting your mind in the same direction as the team's is an important first step. It should also be comforting to know that all of the caregivers are going to work together to help you return to your home setting or appropriate new home setting where the quality of your life including your physical, emotional, and psychosocial well-being will be maximized. While the entire team will work with you to achieve that goal they will not do the work for you.

The Administrator (ADM)

Every skilled nursing facility must have an acting administrator. The facility will literally hang a framed license on the wall somewhere in public view so you can see who is serving in that role. The administrator is a licensed healthcare professional responsible for the overall running of the skilled nursing facility. The non-nursing professionals or departments, usually including the medical director, social work, activities, housekeeping, laundry, business office manager, building maintenance, purchasing, and the dining/kitchen professionals, all report directly to the administrator. In larger organizations there may be an assistant administrator and/or administrator in training on the team. There is always a leader from this team available to support the non-clinical staff, residents, and families.

The Director of Nursing (DON)

The director of nursing is the senior, most clinical leader of the nursing department. And while you may not meet or see this person, it's good to know that he or she exists should you have any questions or concerns about the care that you are receiving. You are more than likely going to interact with a licensed practical nurse or a registered nurse who will do a comprehensive assessment of you upon admission. I'm also going to let you know that this is not the only person who is going to do a comprehensive assessment on you upon admission, and this may start to feel very repetitive and leave you wondering if anyone in the skilled nursing facility even talks to one another. I assure you not only do they talk to one another, but they work intentionally to design a plan of care to meet all of your care needs from medications, food preferences, activities you like to do for fun, and passions which engage your psychosocial needs beyond just your physical needs. They care about your moods, emotions, and desire for religious and spiritual practices - holistic person-centered care is in the very fabric of the industry. So on this first day and maybe sometimes on the second day of arrival you may be getting asked the same question by multiple caregivers as each one of them is working to gather information from a different perspective in order to build their piece of your comprehensive, whole person care plan. The Director is ultimately responsible for the execution and outcomes of your whole person plan. As the title implies, they are directing and not one of the actors you might see "on stage". If something is not going right, or the actors appear to have missed their "lines", talk to the Director of Nursing. If things are going really great and you want to be sure the staff are recognized for their service, talk to the Director of Nursing. In both cases they want to hear from you.

Physical, Occupational, and Speech Therapy

Most people who enter skilled nursing facilities will need the daily skilled services of a physical therapist. Physical therapists focus on how you move. Movement in bed and out of bed, on and off chairs, in and out of a car, up and down stairs, to and from different locations, in your room in and out of your home, and accessing the community. Remember when I asked you to think about your normal daily activity and how and when you complete certain tasks if you use assistive devices? That information is gold to a physical therapist. So if you have brought your card or a copy of your card you'll be able to share that with them, and they will immediately understand what your normal level of function was, and they will start from there in formulating a plan to get you back to that level of function. Their plan will include exercise, range of motion, strength endurance, use of devices, and teaching you how to do your old activities using new habits and new skills.

In addition to the physical therapist, most patients who enter a skilled nursing facility will require the skilled services of an occupational therapist. The occupational therapist focuses on your activities of daily living and how you get those done. Activities of daily living include how you bathe and get dressed, brush your teeth, prepare a meal, care for yourself in the shower, get on and off a toilet, and manage clothing and hygiene. There is some overlap between occupational and physical therapy since there is movement required in completing the activities of daily living. Sometimes these therapists will actually work with you together.

You may also be receiving skilled therapy from a speech language pathologist. These professionals focus on communication, how you formulate and express speech, and address any difficulty you or your loved one may be having with swallowing both food and liquid.

These are some of the key members of the team; there are also dieticians, food service directors, activities coordinators, housekeeping, laundry, and environmental services staff. Their role in creating an environment where you are your loved one should not be overlooked or minimized. My aunt Chum, whose photo graces the cover of this book, chose her assisted living location because of the food service director. It was a delightful surprise while on tour to bump into an old familiar face. Just a few years prior this person had been driving the van that took my aunt on weekly shopping trips. For the next 18 months my aunt was never happier than when she had a visit, or special meal, courtesy of the food service director. *There are dozens of heroes who come to work in nursing homes every day. Be sure to thank each of them when you see them.*

Medical Directors and Skilled Nursing Facility Attending Doctors

If you are wondering who is calling the shots, the answers are here. While at the skilled nursing facility (SNF) your care will be directed by a physician, a nurse practitioner, or a physician's assistant with credentials to practice at that skilled nursing facility. This will not be your primary care doctor whom you see when you are at "home". This will most likely not be a doctor you've ever met before. Like in the hospital where there was coverage by a hospitalist, in the skilled nursing facility local physician practice groups provide services of medical coverage to skilled nursing facilities. Some facilities hire their own dedicated physicians known as SNFists. Those terms might sound like a new type of illness, especially when the nurses tell you they will see if your SNFists are coming in today!

The covering physician in the skilled nursing facility will review the information that the hospital doctor has sent to them at the time of your transfer. Unfortunately, during times of transition information can be lost in communication. This is why I encourage patients or their loved ones to advocate and get a complete copy of the medication orders, the diet orders, and the activity orders and take another copy of that advance directive from the refrigerator with you in your hand when you move from the hospital to a skilled rehabilitation center.

Overall, this is a great plan for effective care delivery for people moving through the skilled nursing facility as these professionals are highly skilled in caring for very sick people who have left the hospital after having an acute event. So while this is very good for the care team, it may feel awkward to you as a patient to be met by a team of virtual strangers. That's why you have to be your own B.I.T.C.H The information that you are learning and your communication tips and tricks will make you successful at not only surviving this rehab course, but actually thriving while you are in it. Remember, ownership and accountability and advocacy are going to be essential for yourself as the patient, or for a loved one that you may be advocating for you.

Understand the goals and objectives of this care team are to safely and effectively discharge you home or to a new home-like setting in the shortest amount of time needed. They also want you to go home and not be readmitted to a hospital. Predicting a date, using an estimate of how many days you need to stay in the SNF before going home, will be used to set an estimated discharge date. The SNF team is going to work to set this point as a date in time. Knowing this is important as you come into the rehab setting so that the questions you ask and the effort you put forth each day in your rehabilitation course is all directed at this end goal of going home and staying there.

The person or people who are quarterbacking this journey as you move through the skilled nursing facility is reading this book. While the care team in the skilled nursing facility cares deeply about your health outcomes, no one cares more than you, no one is going to own every detail more than you, and you should not be waiting around and expecting someone else to lead the coordination, communication, and collaboration of your care needs. Keep in mind these caregivers come into a very busy, institutional environment where they have been outnumbered with more patients than there is time in the day for them to function as a sole advocate. Expecting them to keep all of your details top of mind and separated from the details of 10 or 15 other equally complex, equally important human lives is unrealistic. If you think about that, and then watch the job that they do every day, you'll step back and realize that you're being cared for by some very amazing human beings. Having said all that, the job of quarterback is solely the responsibility of yourself or your advocate so keep reading!

Administrator: A licensed healthcare professional responsible for the overall running of the skilled nursing facility. The non-nursing professionals or departments usually including the medical director, social workers, activities, housekeeping, laundry, business office manager, building maintenance, purchasing, and the dining/kitchen professionals report directly to the administrator. In larger organizations there may be an assistant administrator and/or administrator in training on the team. There is always a leadership person from this team available to support the non-clinical staff, residents, and families.

Director of Nursing: A licensed registered nurse who is responsible for the overall clinical outcomes of the skilled nursing facility. All the nursing staff including RNs, LPNs, CNAs, Medication Techs, along with some roles you might not see which are clinical specialties and include wound care, infection preventionists, quality assurance, and in some organizations the rehab director and their teams. These licensed and certified professionals all report to the Director of Nursing. In larger facilities the DON may have one or more assistant DONs in addition to shift supervisors. There is always a leadership person from this team available when needed to support the clinical staff, residents, or families.

Social Services or Case Manager: Who you contact if you have questions about your insurance coverage, plan of care in the SNF, or the plan for getting back home called the discharge plan, home care services, community resources, or any other question regarding the services which are available in the SNF.

> **Charge Nurse or Shift Supervisor**: Ask for this person if you or your loved one have any concerns about the care received by your nurse or nursing assistants including meals, snacks, medications, skin care, bathing needs, restrictions on activities (in and out of the room), or how you are moving in and around your room.

The Rules and Regulations You Want to Know When Receiving Services in a Skilled Nursing Facility

If you or one of your loved ones are receiving care from a skilled nursing facility, it's important for you to have a good understanding of both how the business operations of the institution are generally managed in order to demonstrate compliance with the regulatory environment which governs the industry. This is not a profession you get into if you can't live by and demonstrate full cooperation with hundreds of rules, all at the same time.

Skilled nursing facilities are licensed by state agencies within each of the states in which they function. However, each facility must operate in compliance with a set of federal regulations put forth for all skilled nursing and long-term care facilities nationwide in the United States. Facilities are inspected annually and as needed following a complaint. These "annual" inspections can happen no sooner than nine months from the prior inspection and shouldn't be any longer than 15 months from that prior inspection. Annual inspections are always unannounced to the provider. There may be a 6-month period of time where the annual inspection is thought to occur, but the exact day, date, and time is a surprise!

The results of these inspections are available for the public to see on carecompare.com and are required to be posted in a visible public place inside the institution. In addition to annual state inspections, there is an ombudsman's office in every state where you can seek advice or guidance on a complaint that you might have around the quality of care you or your loved one may be receiving. The ombudsman, upon receiving a complaint, will do an investigation at the facility also known as a "complaint driven inspection". These inspections are known as complaint investigations or complaint surveys to the SNF professional.

It's good to know that this structure is in place within every state; however, it is not what I recommend as your first line of problem solving or conflict resolution. As I have mentioned, to be your own B.I.T.C.H requires consistent, clear communication, and as the advocate you are responsible for the coordination of this process. With focus on communication and asking the right questions of the right employees within the skilled nursing facility, you will find yourself a well informed consumer of their services. This should be the best approach to preventing or alleviating any concerns around care delivery.

However, there may be times when an individual staff person yields an unsatisfactory response or is not following through with obtaining the information that you need for care, coordination, and collaboration. In that instance the best approach to take is to move within the leadership system of the skilled nursing facility. The nurse that is assigned to you or your loved one for the day most often reports to a charge nurse who is in charge of the unit for a period of time. Some organizations also have Unit Managers who assume responsibility for the unit around the clock 24/7, and those charge nurses often report to an Assistant Director of Nurses or a Director of Nurses. Larger facilities often have shift supervisors to support the charge nurses and unit managers. Following this chain of command is the best approach for raising a concern and getting a systematic response. It's important to keep in mind that skilled nursing facilities are like small manufacturing plants.

Imagine the challenge of needing to get 100 human beings successfully awakened, bathed, dressed, medicated, fed, and ready for their day all at the same time. In order to successfully balance the needs of the individual with the needs of the institution, systems and procedures are implemented that maximize staff efficiency. When you understand how the systems are running, you can have some empathy and be a little curious about how those systems may be impacting the care delivered to you or your loved one. Following the chain of command with any kind of a concern is the best way to dovetail your needs into the institutional policies and procedures. The people who know those best are the leaders within the clinical team.

Let's say for example you prefer to take a shower at night right before bed. You request this as this is your normal routine at home, and you want to follow that normal routine at home as best as you can. The response from the nursing facility could be something as simple as stating that it's their policy that your particular room number gets a shower on Tuesdays in the morning. This may seem like a ridiculous response to a request to have an evening shower. The organization is staffed the heaviest during the 7:00AM to 3:00PM shift or the 7:00AM to 7:00PM shift. This is because there are three meals during that 12-hour block and a lot of activity of people coming and going consisting of new admissions, discharges, doctor's appointments, physician visits, family visitors, as well as support staff that come to the facility during the daytime hours and demand time and interactions from the staff. There's less staff in the evening time and even less staff in the overnight hours when people are typically sleeping. So, it may require some system's management on the part of a charge nurse to adjust the schedule in order to deliver that bedtime shower for you or your loved one. There would be an effort to individualize the plan of care and deliver that shower in the evening, but there also would be a need for some understanding and empathy should staffing not allow for that extra attention in the shower on a particular night. I mentioned that occupational therapists help teach you how to regain the skills of bathing in the shower, and many times the showers are given by the therapists who support the nursing staff with getting the needs of the patients met. This can often be more challenging in the evening hours when the supportive staff like occupational therapists are not working.

In the unlikely event that you have requested or noted concerns around care, properly communicated them within the leadership of the organization, and still feel that the care needs of yourself or your loved one are not being met, the ombudsman's office is there to support and to investigate whether or not your concerns are in fact representative of non-compliance in care. There are a lot of rules to follow in the skilled nursing facility, and the ombudsman's office will listen to any concerns that you have and perform a proper investigation of the facility to validate if your concerns are out of compliance with the standards set forth by the federal government for provision of care in a skilled nursing facility. You can find more information about this nationwide ombudsman program and your local ombudsman office's contact information on the Internet if you search for an ombudsman program and input your state.

Tips for advocating to SNF leadership or the state ombudsman:

- If you have questions or concerns, always begin with the nurse taking care of yourself or your loved one or speak to the nurse who is in charge for that particular day also known as a charge nurse or shift supervisor. Asking for assistance to understand the plan of care or current situation is a perfect conversation to have with a shift supervisor or the director of nurses. By following the advice in this book, you will have been making clear communications to the skilled nursing facility with some regular pattern, and you should have clear data with which to use in your conversations around any care concerns.

- It will be necessary for you to understand that your loved one is living in an institution whose effectiveness requires

---

organization-wide policies and procedures. Many times, when you ask a staff member a direct question they may begin an answer about yourself or your loved one which is reflecting the company's policy or procedure on how things are done. Understand they are running these organizations following regulatory guidelines and in order to ensure that those regulatory guidelines are met. The organization must write down their instructions, known as a policy, with details for each member of the workforce to follow, known as procedures. What's interesting for me as an advocate is that many of these regulatory rules, policies, and procedures contradict one another, and it's often difficult to figure out which policy is trumping the other. For example, residents are supposed to have a personalized plan of care, meaning that they should be able to eat at whatever time they wish to eat. At the same time the state agency is monitoring for the hours which pass in between meals. Should a resident choose to fast, for example, intermittently for 12 hours or 14 hours before having a meal, they should be entitled to choose such meal programming. Such instructions can be documented in their plan of care. The whole industry focuses on resident centered plans of care. However, in many instances the staff might inform the patient that they have to eat at certain times of day because that's the time when they typically serve their meals. I bring up this simple example to help illustrate the tension which exists in care settings where personalized care is desired and sought after by everyone who enters the facility, and yet the staff and staffing ratios are simply not equipped to handle individualized personalized care. So when possible, we convince patients to eat at the same time and go to bed at the same time for the convenience, efficiency, and effectiveness of the organizational function.

Your role is to advocate for a single person who has come to a facility at one point in time and you are trying to get the individual care needs of your loved one met. Choose to advocate on what is most important and compromise when possible.

- Determine critical requests from those "nice to haves". At the end of the day, the care needs of yourself or your loved one is a top priority, and it is fantastic that you're here to advocate for them. This tip encourages you to be reasonable with the requests that you make of the staff. They are working around the clock to meet the care needs of all of the members of the population that they serve, oftentimes without proper time for meal breaks or even bathroom breaks over the course of every 8, 10, or 12 hour shift. When you are feeling disappointed, try to take a step back and look at the operations of the facility as a whole, and not any one individual day. Ask yourself if your expectations of the staff are more than you would expect from yourself as a caregiver? We are all human after all.

- Visit at different times of the day and speak with the staff each time you visit. Request the same staff members take care of your loved one for consistency whenever possible.

- Speak up if you see a pattern of care concerns that puts your loved one, and maybe other members of the community, in jeopardy. That's the time to raise your concern to either the leadership within the skilled nursing facility including the director of nurses or the administrator. If this step gets no resolution to the problem you could certainly speak with the state ombudsman as mentioned prior.

Leading the Coordination, Collaboration, and Communication of Your Health Plan Benefits

Ever feel frustrated trying to understand your health plan benefits, what's covered, and why something might not be covered? You are NOT alone! You will not learn everything about the complexities of health plans in this section, but you will gain enough basic knowledge to ask meaningful questions and be empowered to coordinate, collaborate, and communicate your needs (the "C" in B.I.T.C.H.). This section will review the basics of the two major sources of health insurance coverage for adults over 65 and offer some tips along the way. This section offers a bit more content, and you may need to read it a couple of times to get the lessons you need.

You may not be sure what coverage you or your loved one has. The good news is, in every institution where you seek healthcare services, there are individuals whose job it is to speak to your health plan (think of them as internal advocates). If you are advocating for someone else, ask them to get all of the insurance cards they have in their wallets out. It is possible to have a card and find out that the plan was changed and your loved one no longer has that coverage. Insurance is confusing, the commercials make it sound easy, and our loved ones call those 800 numbers and make changes they don't understand. By calling the numbers on the back of those cards, you can get to a person who can verify your coverage, and help you to know which type of insurance, typically Medicare or Managed Medicare, your loved one has.

It helps to know a little bit more about the organizations in the healthcare system that are paying for healthcare delivery today in 2023. I will refer to them simply as Payers. These organizations have evolved in American history from government programs to contracts into private entities. In 1965, the Social Security Act was amended to include Medicare benefits for Americans who are over 65 years of age and needed insurance coverage for healthcare. The management of this benefit has rested solely with government agencies up until the mid-

1990s when an emerging trend resulted in private sector insurance companies taking on Managed Medicare programs.

In Traditional Medicare insurance, there is a portion of your benefits for when you need hospital care, and there is a portion of your benefits for when you need to see a doctor in the community or receive outpatient services. When you are sick and require admission to a hospital for more than three nights, there are benefits referred to as your "skilled benefit" which can give paid time in a skilled nursing facility to receive skilled nursing or skilled therapy services which were necessary and related to the reason that you were admitted to the hospital. This is what's known as your skilled benefit, and there is a maximum of 100 days which can be paid under the skilled benefit for any one benefit period. There are complex rules around earning new benefit periods which will not be covered here. The basic premise of Medicare is to provide insurance for someone over 65 who gets sick, needs to go to the hospital, or stays for at least three nights as an inpatient in the hospital. Then, should that person require follow up skilled services, they could receive those services in a skilled nursing facility.

These services are not simply custodial in nature; they require the skill of a licensed registered nurse or a licensed physical, occupational, or speech therapist on a daily basis. For nursing, daily means every day or seven days a week. For therapy, daily means five days out of seven in a week. Administering this benefit and monitoring the benefit for appropriate utilization ensuring no fraud or abuse takes place is an expensive, essential part of the US government compliance program. Frankly, I'm not sure how good our government is at administering benefits over time. They contract with private companies to do ongoing contract work to oversee the administration of these benefits. It makes sense that private insurance companies who were already building infrastructure and systems to administer insurance funding to people under 65 could be successful at applying it to populations of

Americans over 65 and effectively improve the quality of the care while saving costs along the way. This was the idea behind the introduction of Managed Medicare programs in the mid-1990s. The hypothesis that management would be more successful when contracted to other organizations was yet to be proven.

Today, the number of Americans enrolling in the Managed Medicare program has grown significantly over the past decade. While there appears to be additional benefits and some reduction in cost to each individual when electing a Managed Medicare program, there is some additional oversight that comes with human capital tightly managing costs for an organization at large. What this means for you as an individual is that when you need services, they're going to have to be authorized by another individual, typically a nurse called a "case manager" who works for the managed care company. As I've pointed out clearly in this book, they are in business to make money and drive down costs of care while at the same time providing high quality services that you are satisfied with. That balancing act is tricky, and you don't want to be the one on the short end of the stick- so to speak.

For all of the advantages that managed care might offer, there are disadvantages that have been observed. Since providers will not provide free care nor should we expect them to, they will require the managed care company to authorize services in advance. You will hear sentences said to you like, "your insurance company has authorized seven days of skilled services" after which you will have to go home unless they authorize an extension. These kinds of comments can induce a lot of stress on the family. Those of us who work in healthcare often refer to managed care as disadvantaged care because the pressure to get home is so intense it definitely feels at times that they are rushing you through the system at a pace that you're not sure you can keep up with.

In contrast, Traditional Medicare, which certainly has requirements for meeting program guidelines, comes with less pressure and gives the provider the responsibility to assure that the services you're receiving require and meet the skilled level of care requirements on a daily basis. When it is anticipated that you will no longer meet the skilled level of care requirements, a notice of advanced beneficiary non-coverage will be issued to you at least 48 hours in advance of your last covered day in the program. Since the skilled services are being administered by the nursing home and documented by the nursing home under their own compliance program, there is more confidence and assurance that all of your skilled needs are taken into consideration following program guidelines before discharge to home is set. Traditional Medicare focuses on guidelines of the skilled program over cost savings. Over time, the US government is introducing small bonus programs for skilled nursing providers which will take into account their overall cost to the Medicare program, and so at some point in the future skilled nursing providers may also start to put a little bit more focus and attention on getting you home quicker.

From my experience I have concluded there are more benefits to staying in a Traditional Medicare program. Working directly with the SNF provider I found more control over the exact day and time that you will transition to home, and more coordination of that transition. The skilled nursing provider also has a greater sense of accountability to you since you are the only two parties making the decision around when is best for a discharge to home transition event. In my opinion, under Managed Medicare when the insurance company gets in the middle, the skilled nursing provider "puts their hands up" as if the decision is out of their control, and they don't share as much accountability in the decision.

The whole premise behind this book is to improve your education about the healthcare system so you can better advocate for yourself or your loved one as you move through it. So as I mentioned, not only is it important for the provider of care to know who's paying for the services that they are about to render, it's also important that you know what benefits you have either Traditional Medicare or Managed

Medicare. Once you have determined who the primary payer is, you should refer to the list of tips specific to those payers which will be listed at the end of this chapter. Keep in mind that the provider of services, simplified to the provider, wants to make sure they receive prompt payment as well as ensuring that you and the patient receive effective care. Keeping up to date information on your insurance coverage in the hands of your providers, makes it easier for them to get paid for the services they provide to you.

Tips for Traditional Medicare Beneficiaries

- Keep track of how many days of skilled service you or your loved one has received. Inpatient census is determined by where you or your loved one sleeps each day at midnight. If you have transitioned from a hospital to a skilled nursing facility and you arrive before midnight, that day will be counted as one of your skilled Medicare days.

- Confirm the dates you were admitted to the hospital. Following a three-night hospital inpatient admissions status you are eligible for up to a maximum of 100 days under your Medicare skilled benefit.

- Know what skilled services are required. In order to stay in the skilled nursing facility you must require and receive a daily skill from either the licensed nurses or the skilled therapists. As mentioned earlier in this book, documenting in detail how you or your loved one typically performed activities of daily living prior to the hospitalization is essential. Medicare pays for skilled services to be provided as long as you or your loved one are making reasonable progress towards this prior level of function. As an advocate you are going to want to speak to this portion of the regulation when you are asking for more time in a skilled nursing facility in order to achieve certain functional goals prior to discharge. Additionally, changes in your health status which occur as a result of the condition which resulted in hospitalization can be considered a skilled service and require observation and assessment from a nurse or evaluation and management from a nurse. These complications which arise while in the skilled nursing facility may prolong your skilled nursing benefits.

- Medicare Part A covers 100% of the first 20 days in a skilled nursing facility. On the 21st day, you or your loved one will be responsible for a copayment for every day thereafter. In 2023 the copayment is 200 dollars per day, this rate can go up every year. This is why it's important to keep track of which day of your Medicare Part A stay you are currently on and be aware of when your copayment responsibilities will begin. If you have a secondary insurance carrier, they may pay the copayment starting on day 21 for you. These are important questions that you should ask and know prior to and while receiving services in a skilled nursing facility.

- Ask when the facility anticipates discharge to home or denial of skilled benefits. The skilled nursing facility will have either set a discharge date for home which they can communicate to you, or they may have simply estimated that you or your loved one needs an additional number of weeks of inpatient rehab. *You should be asking this question at least three times a week when visiting the facility.* If the team believes that a home discharge is safe, they will estimate the number of weeks it's going to take for your loved one to achieve the functional goals necessary to discharge home safely. As long as your loved one is making progress towards those goals, Medicare will pay for your services. If your loved one fails to make progress and the facility needs to issue a denial letter, you will be notified. For many families the letter of non-coverage provokes emotion, fear, and disappointment with the healthcare system. At this time when a letter of non-coverage is delivered to you, the reality sets in that your loved one may not be getting any better and may need to go home with additional support and care from family members - maybe even yourself. We will talk more about caregiver burden and some tips for caregivers later in this book.

This is a complicated portion of the Medicare coverage regulations and if you have a complex situation, you may need to seek some additional help from the facility social worker, case manager, or Director of Nursing. I have some additional resources you might find helpful on my website. If the skilled nursing facility believes that you or your loved one no longer meet the requirements of daily skilled services, they will communicate this decision to you in writing through what's called a "notice of Medicare no coverage". This letter will be issued at least 48 hours prior to their last anticipated cover day from Medicare. You have a right to appeal this decision should you believe that additional skilled services are required by you or your loved one. The nursing home will notify you of your right to appeal the decision and actually assist you in completing the paperwork. A local agency under contract to review these cases will render a decision within 48 hours. Should they decide in your favor, the nursing home will continue to bill Medicare for those skilled services for a finite period of time. Typically, a few days to a week.

At the end of that time, the SNF will once again determine if skilled services are required or should be denied. If the agency supports the decision to deny the skilled benefit, then you or your loved one would need to pay privately for those additional days that you were in the skilled nursing facility waiting for the appeal decision to be rendered. I have appealed these decisions twice for personal family members and both times had the appeal supported. In each situation my loved one received a few more days of skilled services. I recommend that if you have concerns about the needs of your loved one being skilled and disagree with the recommendation to deny services, and you can afford the payment of the few days it might cost you, that you follow the appeal process.

Tips for Managed Medicare Beneficiaries

- Your managed care company may not require a three-night inpatient stay in the hospital to access this benefit.
- Find out the name and contact information of the case manager who was working inside the provider setting, in this case a skilled nursing facility. Your insurance company will not communicate directly with you; they will communicate through the provider's designated case manager who often is a licensed nurse who does not provide direct care to you. They organize the information they receive from the nurses who do care for you and the therapists who treat you in order to provide a summary of how you are doing to your insurance company.
- Ask how many days the insurance company has authorized skilled services to be received for. Ask when the next update to the insurance company is requested to be provided.
- Find out the name and phone number of the case manager that your insurance company has assigned to do the communication to the skilled nursing facility, and although you will not be communicating directly with the insurance company, in most cases this is important to have in case the provider case manager is unavailable and you have questions for the insurance company you want to get directly. Don't wait until you need the information to get the information -

seek this out proactively upon arrival to the skilled nursing facility.

- Managed Medicare companies do not need to wait until you no longer need skilled services to issue a denial letter and send you home. Manage Medicare companies will oftentimes provide skilled services to you in your home, and sometimes this may be very agreeable to you or your loved one. Other times this may feel very rushed.

- You have the right to appeal any decisions around a denial. This is called an advanced beneficiary notice of non-coverage. Medicare notice of non-coverage letters and they are supposed to be issued 48 hours before your last cover day of services. Managed Medicare companies are notorious for issuing denial letters in less than 48 hours, or back-date the letter.

- When a decision is made to deny your benefits the provider and health plan are required to provide an advanced notice. Know the process and speak up when it's not being followed.

As you progress physically, mentally, emotionally, and spiritually through the course of your rehabilitation stay, continue to ask questions. Continue to advocate for yourself, keeping an eye on your own goals and thinking about how to achieve those goals in your prior home setting realistically. Take a close look at your prior activities of daily living worksheet and ask yourself where you are physically today and how much of a gap exists between where you are today and where you were prior to your "Oh Sh*t" moment.

The care team is helping you to determine and set realistic and achievable goals. During the course of your rehab stay you will meet with your team of care providers and your family to discuss the discharge plan and even set a projected date for transitioning back home. While this process took a few sentences for me to describe, you may find this process is actually quite hurried in the care setting. The total duration of time that seniors are spending in short stay rehabilitation programs is getting shorter and shorter every year with the average length of stay being around 20 days for Traditional Medicare payers and around 14 days for Managed care payers. It may feel that the minute you get settled into rehab someone is packing you up and sending you back home, so prepare for that feeling.

Keep your worksheets in mind and complete them before you transition to your next care setting or even back in your prior home setting. With hard work, advocacy, and leveraging the services from the various exceptional professionals that you have met along your journey in the healthcare system, you can achieve your goals of going back home. The chosen care setting or home setting that you transition to most likely will still require that you leverage some services from within your home or within your community, and the advocacy skills that you've learned throughout this book will also serve you in that setting.

When Your Needs Change and the Skilled Nursing Facility May Not Be the Right Place to Be: Transitioning Back to an Emergency Department or Hospital

The whole premise behind skilled nursing facilities is that they provide a valuable service to the healthcare system along a usual and predictable course of recovery. Modern medicine has given us the knowledge to anticipate normal recovery from illness, and so the care providers in the skilled nursing facility are able to anticipate a usual course of recovery and healing based on the known diagnosis that you or your loved one has experienced. Unfortunately, there are times when a new diagnosis or unexpected outcome of a certain illness is noted by the caregivers at the skilled nursing facility. When the diagnosis that they are treating becomes unknown, they have a responsibility and a necessity to get support in determining what new condition you or your loved one might be experiencing. There are lots of little things that change in the course of your recovery and most will be observed and treated right in the SNF. Sometimes bigger changes result in an unexpected clinical presentation of yourself or your loved one, and you may need to go back to the hospital for testing and or treatment.

In the event that you or your loved one presents with unexpected clinical findings or an urgent change in condition which cannot be understood or explained given your current diagnosis, you may find that you need to transition back to a hospital setting. Going back to the hospital setting may be necessary in order to appropriately diagnose and establish a treatment plan for the new condition presenting itself. There are actually many complications of health conditions and illnesses that skilled nursing facilities can effectively diagnose and treat right in the skilled nursing facility without the need to return to an acute hospital setting. These situations look similar to your first "Oh Sh*t" moment in that you will go back to the emergency department. Here, the expertise and medical equipment is utilized to quickly and effectively diagnose the new condition, and then based on the treatment plan for that condition determine if you can return to the skilled nursing facility to return to receive appropriate treatment. Keep in mind that skilled nursing facilities do not provide all medical services, and they do not have access to all medical diagnostic equipment. A lot of progress has been made using technology and telehealth visits that makes it possible for a physician to do an assessment while you or your loved ones stay in the skilled nursing facility. If this virtual assessment determines that additional testing is needed, and that testing is not able to be done remotely in the skilled nursing facility, transfer to an emergency department may be necessary. If that happens to you or your loved one, refer back to the chapter on heading to the ED/ hospital.

As the person or advocate for the person in the SNF setting with a change in condition you may feel that the SNF is waiting too long to "send you back to the ER or hospital". Emergency departments are very busy, often "overflowing" with people awaiting evaluations, admission space, etc. Treatment provided to you utilizing nursing and medical services in place at the SNF may be the best option for you given your condition and the conditions in the local community emergency department. Additionally, the SNF staff are looking to reduce the number of people they send back to the hospital to both lower the overall cost of care and impact their own Medicare reimbursement as there is a penalty imposed for sending someone back to the hospital unnecessarily. Collecting data and analyzing it takes time to make that determination.

The United States Centers for Medicare and Medicaid Services implemented a penalty program designed to motivate the cooperation of many providers of healthcare within the system to reduce unnecessary returns to hospital admissions. This focus places a lot of pressure on operators of skilled nursing facilities to carefully scrutinize every transfer to the hospital or to the emergency department to make sure that it is clinically necessary to do so. This translates into improved care collaboration and communication between hospitals, skilled nursing professionals, and home health providers.

As the person in the center of that system you should know that these providers are working tirelessly to build systems which prevent unnecessary return to the hospital or emergency department "events". What does this mean for you as the person in the middle of the system? You may see an increased use of telehealth. Even if you are feeling like you want or need to go back to the hospital, there will be an effort made to apply appropriate diagnostic and assessment techniques to you to determine the cause of whatever change in clinical condition is being noted. This effort is focused on keeping you in the skilled nursing facility and treating whatever that new condition is in the skilled nursing facility whenever possible.

A simple example might be that a patient enters the skilled nursing facility for rehabilitation following a fall with fractured a hip and pelvis, and a week into the skilled nursing facility stay develops a fever and cough. The skilled nursing facility will have the on-call physician, or a telehealth physician do a virtual visit of the patient. They will order routine lab work as well as diagnostic work to evaluate the chest for congestion like a chest X-ray. When possible, they will treat with oral or IV antibiotics to combat any infection that may have been noted.

There are several types of acute illnesses which arise as a complication due to just being sick and having your normal body rhythms impacted by a change in one's ability to function physically, mentally, and based on medical conditions biochemically. The example above of an upper respiratory infection or even bronchitis and pneumonia, bladder infections, skin inflammation, or other minor conditions are quite commonly diagnosed and treated in the skilled nursing facility.

This is in contrast to conditions such as sudden onset of major organ function like a heart attack, kidney failure, or gallbladder attack which would require both medical specialists to assist in guiding the diagnosis and treatment of those conditions as well as a more intensive around the clock monitoring and assessment of one's condition in the early days after new onset of major changes in your overall health. In those instances it may be absolutely necessary to return to the hospital and receive the appropriate supportive care because the condition is so new and major that it exceeds the capacity of a skilled nursing facility. Remember, a skilled nursing facility is exceptionally good at taking a known diagnosis with an anticipated treatment plan and monitoring you or your loved one through the course of that treatment plan and alerting your doctor when you or your loved one's condition veers off the expected clinical pathway.

Sometimes a transition back to the emergency department of the hospital is absolutely necessary. In those instances the skilled nursing facility is going to provide all the same information that we highlighted in part one around your medications, your code status or advance directives, your activities of daily living, and how things are usually occurring for you as a reflection of what has happened in the skilled nursing facility.

This may mean that the hospital that is about to get you back is going to see new medications and new functional status since their prior interactions with you. Again, anytime you transition from one institution providing care to another, there's an opportunity for communication to fall through the cracks. Therefore, continuation and coordination of care is interrupted. As an advocate you are going to want to have knowledge of all of the current medications, the current functional status, the current code status, and any specialized needs or treatments so that you can speak to and advocate for those needs upon arriving back at the hospital setting.

Keep in mind that upon arrival back at the hospital the physician in the hospital and the hospitalist on staff are now going to be driving the care of you or your loved one. As an advocate, when you come in with all of the data and you contribute that data to the conversation that you have with the new physician, it helps better equip you to be able to make data-driven decisions and make that decision collaboratively with the hospitalist.

Individually and collectively we all get to determine and have a final say in the care which is given to us. At the end of the day, it is the patient and their family that has the final say in the services that they will receive and the care that will be given to them. I like to say that we pay physicians for the data, but ultimately we make the decisions. When we leverage and utilize the excellent care providers all around us to collect and understand all of the data, we can be the best data-driven decision makers since no one knows you like you know you, and no one will advocate for you the way you shall.

If a trip to the emergency department is needed, you might be able to get checked out and come right back to the skilled nursing facility depending on what care you need. The most effective use of emergency department services from the perspective of the medical staff, specialty staff, and special medical diagnostic testing equipment is to be able to utilize those services to give a quick diagnosis and treatment plan, such that you can rapidly determine if a continued stay in the skilled nursing facility would be possible. As mentioned above, there are some services which are not provided in every skilled nursing facility and some skilled nursing facilities have differentiated themselves in the marketplace by providing higher acute services such as complex IV antibiotics, parenteral or artificial feeding, and even ventilator or tracheostomy care. However, these are not services which are commonly provided at every skilled nursing facility. Depending upon the needs of yourself or your loved one, the emergency department evaluation can quickly tell you if you can return right back to the skilled nursing facility and continue your course of rehab, at the same time healing and recovering from whatever acute illness has crept up along your journey towards home. If necessary, a short stay in the hospital may be a small interruption followed by return to a skilled nursing facility and again ultimately helping complete the course of your journey on route to whatever you call home.

Transitioning Home

There is a cost to coming home for caregivers which may not have been obvious to you before now. The United States healthcare system, value based care models, and emerging payment models are all pushing patients where they want to be: home. And while home is a lovely place for all of us, this puts an incredible strain on the unexpecting caregiver. Whether you are a spouse, partner, daughter, son, niece, nephew, roommate, or friend you have found your way into the role of caregiver. While you have always cared deeply for your person, now it's really different.

As an advocate for a loved one you might find yourself transitioning into a physical caregiver upon the point at which your loved one is ready to come home. You may even find that you have been delivering some physical care, emotional support, and meals in the skilled nursing facility. As you prepare to transition to your loved one home, your job is going to intensify!

In addition to the physical demands of a caregiver, you may be organizing the appointments and driving your loved one to appointments or outpatient therapy sessions. You may also find yourself planning all of the meals, setting up all of the medications, waiting at the door for the visiting nurse staff members to arrive and greeting them, explaining access to them how, they get in and out of the property, and making sure that your loved one is ready to interact with them during their session. There is a cost to coming home for caregivers and it's a big one! Keep in mind that the health insurance company relies on caregivers every day. You should be asking what services your loved one is entitled to under their insurance program and pushing for those services to be delivered in addition to whatever you as a caregiver are willing and able to do.

I know you said for better or worse, in sickness and in health; however, spouses do not have to take on the job of both caregiver and spouse. As an example, when a loved one comes home from the hospital they are in need of services from visiting nurses which may include the care of a certified nursing assistant to help with bathing and dressing. It may include services from a physical therapist to help restore function and strength in ambulation and movement in and out of bed. Oftentimes these needs go overlooked and it's just assumed that the caregiver will fill the gap.

Your job as an advocate is to use your voice, speak up, and make sure that the maximum amount of services the plan will cover are provided in the home for your loved one. This is going to support you as a caregiver and give you some time back for yourself which is desperately needed to prevent burnout.

By burnout I mean feelings of frustration and fatigue that result in a grouchy demeanor. Eventually, over time as a caregiver, if you don't get any break your ability to care for someone else can be compromised and bad outcomes can occur for both of you. The health plan has a vested interest in both of your outcomes if you're on the same plan, so speaking up early and making sure you have as many additional supportive services in the house as possible is important for care for yourself as a caregiver as well as for the long term plan for your loved one. There are many publications, podcasts, resources on caregiver burnout and support. See www.cherylfield.com resources for more.

Preparing for Discharge or Transition Back to a Home and Community Setting

From the moment you enter any emergency department, you or your loved one are wondering when they can get back home. By the time you have spent a few days in a skilled nursing facility, you will already begin to be thinking about what needs to be accomplished functionally and medically in order to achieve a safe discharge back to whatever location you call home. Preparing for this transition home is just as important as it was to prepare for the transition into the emergency department.

As you prepare to transition home from a skilled nursing facility all that same information needs to be updated and brought back with you into the community. In many cases it will be recommended that you continue receiving some services from a visiting nurse in your home to help you manage the transition and any monitoring your doctors recommend. You now want to gather all the same details from the SNF about you, and be prepared to communicate them to the visiting nurses. Although the SNF will share information, remember any accidental omission of information written down could lead to an unwanted outcome for you. Upon this transition home, you or your loved one needs to be ready, be the B.I.T.C.H., which means you need to 1) Be prepared 2) gather Information 3) Take control 4)

Communicate and Collaborate so you get back 5) Home. The same way that you were the voice that brought clearly communicated accurate information into the healthcare system, you are going to be the voice for caring back to those home health agencies that may be supporting you as you come home.

Here are some tips for preparing to transition home:

- Depending upon how long you or your loved one have been out of the home, you may not have given much thought to what's in the refrigerator. Food that has been sitting over 5 days needs to be thrown away prior to returning home. This is easily overlooked in preparation for transition back to the community.

- Plan ahead for healthy meals! Nutrition plays an important role in recovery, and prior to discharge you're going to want to plan ahead for having meals prepared or food brought in and prepared on behalf of yourself or your loved one. Connect with your favorite delivery app like DoorDash or Grubhub or get one of your buddies to prepare some of your favorite dishes and stock the fridge. You just want to make sure that when you arrive home the fridge is clean and empty of all of the old food. Too often we forget exactly how long items have been in the refrigerator and consume foods that are out of date or spoiled which can cause illness and bad reactions.

- You also want to get a list of your current medications from the skilled nursing facility and make sure you know the brand name and the trade name and what that pill looks like. Just like when you were transitioning from home into the hospital setting, it is essential for you to know and understand your current medications.

- Review this list a few times with the nurse or doctor at the SNF. Make sure you know what medications you are on, and why.
- When you get home and you look at your "prior" medication list from before this "Oh Sh*t" moment, you don't want to have any confusion.
- Be aware sometimes as you leave the SNF the doctor there will decide to put you back on the medications you took at home. Ask before you leave if they are planning any changes to the medication list the nurses provided to you. Do not assume! *Do not go back to taking your "old" medications without talking to your doctor.* To thrive in healthcare transitions you must speak up and advocate for your own knowledge and need for information. This is the I.T.C.H. – Information, Transition, Communication needed to get you Home.
- Ask the SNF to send a summary of your stay in the nursing home to your primary care doctor. Your primary care doctor is about to be back in charge!
- Set up an appointment to see your primary care doctor. Sometimes the SNF will do this before you leave. If not, call and set this up for the next 5 days. Remember how I said that you were going to transition back to your primary care doctor for calling the shots? This appointment is essential, and here is why. The physician who is providing orders in the nursing home and your primary care doctor may not agree on the approach to treating your chronic medical conditions. What this means is that once you visit your primary care doctor in the first week or so having been discharged from the skilled nursing facility, he or she is likely to request that you revert back to some of your older medications.

Welcome Home!

Home is a wonderful place to be and if you follow the advice and tips in this book you will be able to safely and effectively navigate the healthcare system on behalf of your loved one or for yourself so that you can spend countless days at home. Be prepared by having the following information easily accessible in places like on your refrigerator, in an envelope behind your front door, or in a shared note on your smartphone which you share with your family or loved one.

Since your primary care doctor may want to change your medications, I recommend that upon transition home you set aside all of your older medications in a container and label them with the date that you set them aside. Then complete your medication chart with all of the medication names, doses, and frequency of usage that you have been taking since leaving the skilled nursing facility. Upon your first visit to your primary care doctor take your "new" list of medications and do a thorough medication reconciliation with your provider. The visiting nurses may also send a nurse into your home one or two days after you have left the skilled nursing facility, and that person will also help you with doing this reconciliation of your medications to make sure that you don't accidentally double up on any medications simply because you do not recognize the names or the purpose of the drug.

My final advice when you do get settled in at home is to update your documents hanging on your refrigerator. Once again you're going to want to update all of the sheets that you need to keep on your refrigerator. You just never know when the next urgent moment will occur, and you will have to reenter the healthcare system. So take a few moments and update your medications, activities of daily living, pain inventory, food or medication allergies, and your advance directives. Evaluate the technology you use to call for help in the event of an emergency and invest in new systems if they were absent before. Now you will be completely prepared in the unwanted event that you need to seek medical assistance again in an institutional setting outside of your own home.

Tips while living at home:

- Keep a complete medication and vaccination list, with dates when last received
- Outline your normal activities of daily living, and any devices you use each day
- Note any limitations or restrictions you have on movement or weight bearing
- Describe any pain you experience, and what helps you most
- Update and share your advance directives
- Have technology/tools for calling for help in case you are not able to get to a phone and call for help
- Bring this information to/from appointments with your primary care doctor

Unfortunately, as humans age, the number of "Oh Sh*t" moments increase. Preparing for the unexpected and having a set of resources like this book will help you over and over. This is not a book you read and donate to a thrift store. The tips and resources can help you or your loved ones navigate their movements through the healthcare system. As a community of growing advocates, each of you as readers may find a tip that others can benefit from, and I invite you to email those suggestions to me so that your insights can help others in future versions of this book.

Resources Section

This book reflects knowledge I have gathered over a 30+ year career in senior care. Below are some of my favorite places I go when I need to learn more details. Additionally, for information on senior care resources including the forms for getting prepared visit my website www.cherylfield.com under the resources tab. I have placed links to items every older American needs including: medication schedules, activities of daily living documents, advance directives by state, incontinence management, safety tips, and more. If you don't see a resource you are looking for email me at info@cherylfield.com.

https://www.medicare.gov/care-compare/?guidedSearch=NursingHome&providerType=NursingHome
https://www.cms.gov/Medicare/Provider-Enrollment-and-Certification/CertificationandComplianc/FSQRS
https://www.ahcancal.org/Pages/default.aspx
https://www.mcknights.com

About the Author

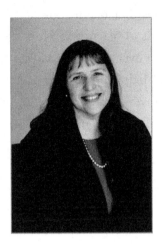

Cheryl Field has 30+ years experience in nursing, specializing in rehabilitation in the post-acute area with a focus on analytics, compliance, quality, and reimbursement. Cheryl has served a variety of roles, including clinical director, VP of Healthcare, Chief Product Officer and most recently as Group Product Leader. Cheryl has written for over 20 years including professional journal articles, online blogs, text book chapters and most recently in the anthology You Can, You Will which became a #1 best seller Internationally. Cheryl has spoken at state and national conventions over 25 years on a variety of healthcare care industry topics. She makes learning complex systems easy with simple analogies, relevant and often personal stories to maximize audience engagement. Cheryl is passionate about advocacy and wants every person to take control of their own destiny when accessing healthcare. Providers are great resources for information, the patient and their family should leverage the information to make their own care decisions. This means providers need to explain the information in an easy to understand and culturally relatable way. To this end Cheryl offers seniors consultation to support their understanding of their current and future health care choices.

Cheryl is certified in Rehabilitation Nursing, and recently achieved certification in machine learning and artificial intelligence from MIT. She holds a Bachelor's of Science in Nursing from the University of Rochester and a Master's of Science in Nursing from Boston College. Cheryl has been married over 30 years to her 3rd grade sweetheart Ted, and has three children Michael, Rebecca and Jennifer. When Cheryl is not working she enjoys gardening, canning, scrapbooking, and spending time with family and friends.

Relevant Awards

Educator of the Year 2008 CT Chapter American College of Health Care Administers;
Pivot award 2020 Point Click Care
Choose to Challenge Award 2021 International Women's Day PointClickCare

Contact information: You can learn more about Cheryl and check out her resource page at www.cherylfield.com or on linked in www.linkedin.com/in/cherylfield1621